Update of Non-Pharmacological Therapy for Heart Failure

Koichiro Kinugawa • Teruhiko Imamura
Editors

Update of Non-Pharmacological Therapy for Heart Failure

Springer

Editors
Koichiro Kinugawa
The Second Department of Internal Medicine
University of Toyama
Toyama, Japan

Teruhiko Imamura
The Second Department of Internal Medicine
University of Toyama
Toyama, Japan

ISBN 978-981-15-4845-1 ISBN 978-981-15-4843-7 (eBook)
https://doi.org/10.1007/978-981-15-4843-7

This Springer imprint is published by the registered company Springer Nature Singapore Pte Ltd.
The registered company address is: 152 Beach Road, #21-01/04 Gateway East, Singapore 189721, Singapore

Contents

Chapter 1
Overview

Koichiro Kinugawa

Abstract In this book, my honorable colleagues dedicated their efforts to describe state-of-the-art technology and strategy for advanced heart failure. We basically focused on non-pharmacological therapy of heart failure, but every non-pharmacological therapy should be added on top of or concomitantly with guideline-directed pharmacological/medical therapy (GDMT). I firstly outline how we implement GDMT to heart failure patients in this chapter, and then miscellaneous matters of non-pharmacological therapy are discussed. References are too many to be cited, and most of them that can be referred in the recent guidelines are omitted from the reference list.

Keywords GDMT · HFrEF · HFpEF · ADHF

1.1 Guideline-Directed Medical Therapy (GDMT) in Chronic Heart Failure (Table 1.1) [1]

Before we initiate therapy for chronic heart failure, we have to know at least one thing, left ventricular ejection fraction (LVEF). Many pharmacological evidences have been established among patients with EF less than 40%, i.e., heart failure with reduced EF (HFrEF), but on the other hand, virtually nothing has known to be effective among patients with EF greater than 50%, i.e., heart failure with preserved EF (HFpEF). According to the limited space, below I will summarize GDMT for HFrEF. First drug evidence of HFrEF has appeared in a not-so-large scale but a randomized place-controlled double blinded manner, i.e., CONSENSUS study in 1987. This study proved the dramatic survival benefit of enalapril, an angiotensin converting enzyme inhibitor (ACEi), and made a landmark trial in cardiovascular medicine. The beneficial effect of ACEi has provoked "angiotensin-ics" resulting in the development of many angiotensin type 1 receptor blockers (ARBs). That was a first approach from bench to bedside in cardiovascular medicine, but we are not

K. Kinugawa (✉)
The Second Department of Internal Medicine, University of Toyama, Toyama, Japan
e-mail: kinugawa-tky@umin.ac.jp

K. Kinugawa, T. Imamura (eds.), *Update of Non-Pharmacological Therapy for Heart Failure*, https://doi.org/10.1007/978-981-15-4843-7_1

Table 1.1 Class of recommendation and level of evidence for drugs used in the treatment of chronic heart failure according to the most recent guidelines

	HFrEF (LVEF < 40%)		HFpEF (LVEF ≥ 50%)
Drugs	Class/level	Special consideration	Class/level
ACEi	I/A		IIb/C
ARB	I/A	Alternative to ACEi, but no superiority proven	IIb/C
ARNI (sacubitril–valsartan)	I/B	Alternative to ACEi/ARB, and superior to ACEi	? (maybe IIb/C)
MRA (spironolactone/ eplerenone)	I/A	Generally recommend to use with RAS inhibitor	IIb/C
Beta blocker (carvedilol/ bisoprolol/metoprolol succinate)	I/A	No class effect proven	IIb/C
If channel inhibitor (ivabradine)	IIa/B	Sinus rhythm, heart rate > 75 bpm, generally recommend in combination with beta blocker	–
SGLT2i (dapagliflozin)	Currently IIa/A (will be I/B)	Currently approved for DM, but will be able to use for non-DM HFrEF/class effect will be proven	–
sGC stimulator (vericiguat)	? (maybe IIa/B)	Yet approved as of early 2020	–
Loop diuretics	I/C		I/C
V_2R antagonist (tolvaptan)	IIa/B	Should be used with loop diuretics	IIa/C

HFrEF heart failure with reduced ejection fraction, *HFpEF* heart failure with preserved ejection fraction, *ACEi* angiotensin converting enzyme inhibitor, *ARB* angiotensin type 1 receptor blocker, *ARNI* angiotensin receptor neprilysin inhibitor, *RAS* renin–angiotensin system, *MRA* mineralocorticoid receptor antagonist, *SGLT2i* sodium-glucose transporter 2 inhibitor, *DM* diabetes mellitus, *sGC* soluble guanylate cyclase, V_2R vasopressin type 2 receptor

lucky enough to grab superior drugs over enalapril so easily. Nevertheless perseverance in the study of renin–angiotensin system (RAS) has finally fructified in angiotensin receptor–neprilysin inhibitor (ARNI) called sacubitril–valsartan, which has demonstrated superiority over enalapril in PARADIGM-HF trial. All developed countries except Japan are now in a trend of switching from ACEi/ARB to ARNI, but ARNI will eventually be approved in mid-2020 also in Japan. ACEi, ARB, or ARNI is not recommended to use in combination. A final product of RAS, aldosterone, binds to mineralocorticoid receptor (MR), and MR antagonists (MRA) such as spironolactone or eplerenone has also been shown to improve outcomes of HFrEF patients. MRA should be used with RAS inhibitor, i.e., one of ACEi, ARB, or ARNI, but usually contraindicated in those who have eGFR below 25.

The most surprising part of drug therapy for HFrEF has prevailed in the late 1990s. Beta blocker has a negative inotropic effect by itself, and therefore has long been considered as a contraindication for systolic dysfunction. Small studies, however, have shown the apparent contradictory benefit of beta blocker among patients with systolic dysfunction, and finally large-scale studies for three beta blockers have demonstrated survival benefit on HFrEF patients. So far, the benefit of beta blocker has never been considered as class effect, and only three drugs, i.e., carvedilol, bisoprolol, metoprolol succinate, are used as proven drugs, although metoprolol succinate is not available in Japan. The beneficial effect of beta blocker is still a mystery, but may partly be explained by reduced heart rate. This concept has been strengthened by the result of SHIFT study, which demonstrated the benefit of sinus node funny current inhibitor, ivabradine among HFrEF patients with relatively fast heart rate even after the introduction of beta blocker. Ivabradine is now approved in Japan as a drug to treat HFrEF with sinus rhythm of heart rate greater than 75 beats per minute.

By the way, why these drugs are effective in the treatment of HFrEF? The most simple explanation is based on the experimental murine model of myocardial infarction. You can easily find left anterior descending artery in the open chest of mouse, and ligation of it results in myocardial infarction. People often choose ischemia-reperfusion model by releasing the ligation after a prespecified time of ischemia. This model consistently associates global hypokinesia and marked eccentric remodeling of left ventricle consisting of thinned wall thickness and enlarged cavity, which is attributable to hypertrophy/apoptotic myocytes within nonischemic area and interstitial fibrosis. Since this model resembles to typical clinical course after human myocardial infarction that results in HFrEF, the above drugs have been tested in this model. Lessons from the murine experimental model and drug effectiveness on human HFrEF are quite consistent, and now we know that HFrEF or eccentric remodeling is a malignant cycle of neurohumoral activation including sympathetic nervous system, RAS cascade especially angiotensin II and aldosterone. Neprilysin deactivates natriuretic peptides that may antagonize the above vicious hormones. The effect of ARNI may be explained by the upregulation of natriuretic peptides that is attributable to neprilysin inhibition by sacbitril, though not fully examined.

1.2 Drugs for Acute Heart Failure (Table 1.2) [1]

Most of the chapters in this book focus on devices/strategies for chronic heart failure, but some of chapters handle devices used in acute cardiogenic shock. In the acute decompensated heart failure (ADHF), conventional treatment using diuretics, vasodilator, and inotropes is a mainstay. Relatively high dose of loop diuretics is still commonly used in Western countries. In contrast, Japanese cardiologists would like to choose vasopressin type 2 receptor antagonists, tolvaptan, in addition to lower dose of loop diuretics. Many randomized controlled studies have already revealed its potent aquaretic effect in the acute heart failure without compromise of renal function, especially in Japanese studies. We published a meta-analysis of 14 randomized studies to confirm the acute efficacy of tolvaptan [2]. Our Japanese guidelines for heart failure recommend tolvaptan as class IIa. Loop diuretics is

Table 1.2 Class of recommendation and level of evidence for drugs used in the treatment of acute heart failure according to the most recent guidelines

Drugs	Special consideration	Class/ level
Loop diuretics		I/C
V_2R antagonist (tolvaptan)	Should be used with loop diuretics	IIa/A
MRA (spironolactone/eplerenone/ potassium canrenoate)	May not indicated for eGFR<25	IIb/C
Nitrates	Multiple form available (oral/intravenous/ sublingual/spray)	I/B
hANP (carperitide)	Avoid long-term usage from dependency	IIa/B
Dobutamine	Eosinophilia is not rare	IIa/C
Dopamine	Renal protection not proven	IIb/A
Norepinephrine	Peripheral hypoperfusion	IIb/B
PDE3i (milrinone/olprinone)	Proarrhythmic especially with renal dysfunction	IIa/A
Beta blocker (landiolol)	Rate control of Af tachycardia	IIa/B
Digitalis	Rate control of Af tachycardia	IIa/C

V_2R vasopressin type 2 receptor, *MRA* mineralocorticoid receptor antagonist, *eGFR* estimated glomerular filtration rate, *hANP* human atrial natriuretic peptide, *PDE3i* phosphodiesterase 3 inhibitor, *Af* atrial fibrillation

often used during chronic phase to control congestion, and tolvaptan is again useful to minimize the dose of loop diuretics and to avoid progressive renal dysfunction and heart failure hospitalizations [3]. Moreover, intravenous form of tolvaptan is now under clinical trial that will be finished in mid-2020. Aggressive decongestion in the setting of ADHF cannot always be done by loop diuretics but concomitant use of intravenous tolvaptan may facilitate decongestion in diuretics-resistance patients.

The failure of ASCEND-HF study [4] has a tremendous impact on the new development of vasodilator. Nesiritide, an intravenous form of B-type natriuretic peptide, has never been thought as ineffective to treat congestive heart failure, but in fail. A sister drug, carperitide, an intravenous atrial natriuretic peptide, is only available in Japan, and still keeps high market share, although no large controlled study supports its benefit. Given that natriuretic peptides are endogenously produced, long-term administration of these drugs may be avoided; otherwise patients lose normal reaction of natriuretic peptide system and as a result are totally dependent upon intravenous drug. Serelaxin, one of a vasodilator, also failed to meet primary endpoint in RELAX-AHF-2 study [5]. Nitrates are therefore the major drug for vasodilation in ADHF. In an emergency room, spray form of nitrate is now common rather than sublingual form. Hydralazine is rarely used in Japan, probably because of its notorious drug-induced lupus, though the incidence in Japanese people has never shown to be high.

There is no recent advance in the field of inotropes, and dobutamine, dopamine, phosphodiesterase (PDE) 3 inhibitors, and norepinephrine are still major actors.

Dobutamine is not uncommonly complicated with eosinophilia. Anecdotal "renal" dose of dopamine has never been established. Long-term usage of norepinephrine often associates peripheral hypoperfusion because of its vasoconstrictive action. Careful monitoring of ventricular arrhythmia is mandatory especially when PDE3 inhibitors are administered to patients with renal dysfunction. Levosimendan is not available in Japan.

In a condition with atrial fibrillation (Af) tachycardia, physicians might want to control heart rate although the precise target rate is yet to be determined in Af patients. As a minimum consensus, heart rate of Af may be controlled below 110 bpm [6], and to do so, intravenous form of beta blocker, landiolol, is widely used in Japan even under systolic dysfunction. Conventional digoxin usage is being less popular after J-Land study [7] because of its slow action on heart rate.

1.3 New Drugs for HFrEF (Table 1.1)

Two new drugs are on the way to approval for HFrEF treatment. One is sodium-glucose transporter 2 inhibitor (SGLT2i), which has originally been introduced as a drug for diabetes. Three cardiovascular outcome trials [8] on SGLT2i have consistently shown the low incidence of heart failure hospitalizations as well as cardiovascular death among type 2 diabetic patients with atherosclerotic cardiovascular disease. Moreover, dapagliflozin has shown the marked improvement in almost all outcomes including all-cause death according to DAPA-HF study [9] conducted among HFrEF patients irrespective of the presence of diabetes. The surprising part of this study lies in equal effectiveness between nondiabetic HFrEF patients and diabetic ones. The precise mechanism how SGLT2i works in nondiabetic patients is yet to be elucidated, but the above classical story of sympathetic nervous system or RAS may not directly be involved in the SGLT2i pathway. However, thanks to the DAPA-HF result, many countries including Japan are now in a process of approving dapagliflozin as a first-line drug for HFrEF.

Above all, the pharmacological evidences have accumulated in HFrEF world, and so far five categories of drugs have been listed as first-line usage, i.e., ACEi/ARB, ARNI, beta blocker, MRA, and SGLT2i. VICTORIA study [10], which has tested the effect of soluble guanylate cyclase (sGC) stimulator, vericiguat, among patients with HFrEF, has revently been reported to improve prognosis among HFrEF patients. sGC stimulator is originally developed as a potent pulmonary vasodilator to treat pulmonary artery hypertension (PAH), but some people have considered it effective in the treatment of postcapillary pulmonary hypertension due to left heart disease. Vericiguat is a sister drug of riociguat that has already been approved for PAH, and has been tested in HFrEF and HFpEF with or without elevated pulmonary vascular resistance. VICTORIA study has enrolled HFrEF patients irrespective of the presence of pulmonary hypertension, and may make the sixth first-line drug. Other mechanisms than vasodilatory action of vericiguat may involve elevated cGMP in cardiac myocyte, but it is totally unknown how elevated intracellular cGMP in cardiac myocyte works and whether such pathway leads to improved outcome of HFrEF.

The efficacy has yet to be proved, but oral myosin activator, omecamtiv mecarvil is now tested in phase III GALACTIC-HF trial (ClinicalTrials.gov Identifier: NCT02678923). This is a new category drug if it shows the survival benefit, since every other drug in GDMT somehow lowers blood pressure or even lowers systolic function but this drug rather increases blood pressure by way of improvement of systolic function. That kind of positive inotropic concept once denied in PROMISE study [11] that tested PDE 3 inhibitor, milrinone, in the long term. If omecamtiv mecarvil will show the benefit, it will change the concept dominating the treatment of HFrEF patients.

Table 1.3 List of non-pharmacological therapy for heart failure

Device/strategy	Major indication	Chapters to refer
CRT/CRT-D	HFrEF with wide QRS	Chap. 3
PV isolation	HFrEF with Af	
LV plasty (SAVE, Dor)	ICM with aneurysm	Chap. 9
AVR (surgical/TAVI)	Severe AS	
MVP/MVR (surgical/MitraClip/TMVr)	Severe MR (degenerative/functional)	Chaps. 8 and 9
IASD	HFpEF with elevated PAWP	
Cardiac rehabilitation	Every HF patient	Chap. 5
NPPV (CPAP/BiPAP/ASV)	Acute pulmonary edema/SAS/long-term congestion	Chap. 4
Multidisciplinary approach	Every HF patient	Chap. 5
Home monitoring (CardioMems/telemonitoring)	Frequent flyer	Chap. 2
Temporary MCS (IABP/ECMO/Impella/extracorporeal VAD)	Cardiogenic shock	Chaps. 6 and 7
Durable MCS (implantable LVAD)	Profile 2–4, modifier A	Chap. 10
Heart transplantation	Stage D w/o exclusion criteria	Chap. 11
Cardiac regeneration therapy	?	Chap. 12

CRT(D) cardiac resynchronization therapy (with implantable cardioverter/defibrillator), *HFrEF* heart failure with reduced ejection fraction, *PV* pulmonary vein, *Af* atrial fibrillation, *LV* left ventricle, *ICM* ischemic cardiomyopathy, *AVR* aortic valve replacement, *TAVI* transcatheter aortic valve implantation, *AS* aortic stenosis, *MVP(R)* mitral valve replacement (repair), *TMVr* transcatheter mitral valve replacement, *MR* mitral regurgitation, *IASD* intra-atrial shunt device, *HFpEF* heart failure with preserved ejection fraction, *PAWP* pulmonary artery wedge pressure, *NPPV* non-invasive positive airway pressure, *CPAP* continuous positive airway pressure, *ASV* adaptive servo ventilation, *SAS* sleep apnea syndrome, *MCS* mechanical circulatory support, *IABP* intra-aortic balloon pump, *ECMO* extracorporeal membrane oxygenation, *(L)VAD* (left) ventricular assist device

1.4 Outline of Non-pharmacological Therapy for Heart Failure (Table 1.3)

Most of non-pharmacological therapy has taken it granted well-treated by GDMT and largely been implemented to HFrEF patients. Table 1.3 summarizes the list of non-pharmacological therapy for heart failure patients. Some of them are performed by cardiac surgeons only, but many of them are now increasingly executed by cardiologists with the help of surgeons. The trend of pursuing noninvasiveness results in marked advancement of catheter-based therapeutic options as listed in this table. The therapeutic modality discussed in the late chapters are also shown in Table 1.3. Figure 1.1 summarizes when to indicate each device along with the stage of heart failure in order to integrate several devices during the clinical course of patients.

Here I will briefly mention other important modalities to save heart failure patients. Af is a common complication of heart failure, and one of factors relates to malignant cycle of failing heart. Recently, CASTLE-AF study [12] revealed that pulmonary vein isolation by catheter ablation was superior to medical treatment among HFrEF patients with Af. Af ablation may be increasingly popular in HFrEF management.

Many of the elderly aortic stenosis (AS) patients who are not indicated for surgical aortic valve replacement (AVR) now receive transcatheter aortic valve implantation (TAVI). Recent data from PARTNER 3 [13] showed that patients at low risk of

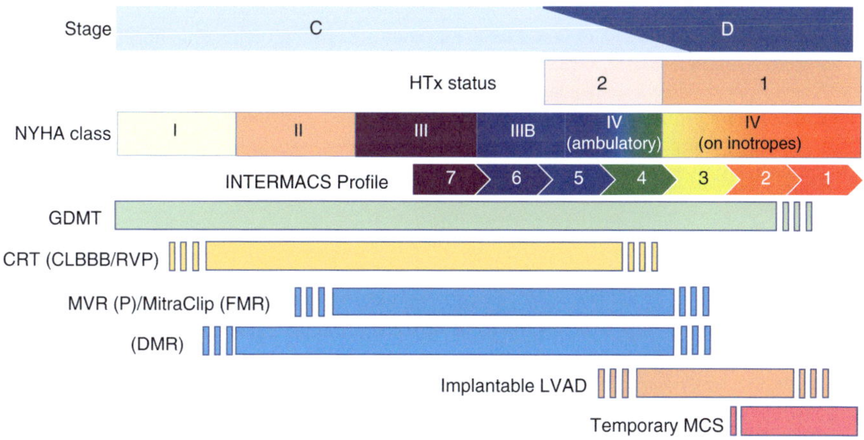

Fig. 1.1 Indication for device/MCS therapy in advanced heart failure. The comparison among Stage classification (C to D), HTx listing status (1 or 2), NYHA functional class (I to IV), INTERMACS profiles (7 to 1) is shown. Medical therapy is always mandatory, but if symptoms persist several devices may be indicated at the appropriate time as shown. *MCS* mechanical circulatory support, *HTx* heart transplantation, *GDMT* guideline-directed medical therapy, *CRT* cardiac resynchronization therapy, CLBBB, complete left bundle branch block; *RVP* right ventricular pacing, MVR(P), mitral valve replacement (repair); F(D)MR, functional (degenerative) mitral regurgitation; *LVAD* left ventricular assist device

open heart surgery rather enjoyed better outcome by TAVI than surgical AVR, and indication for TAVI may be changed in the near future.

Another important device not discussed in the late chapters is intra-atrial shunt device (IASD), which is under phase III study named REDUCE LAP-HF II trial (ClinicalTrials.gov Identifier: NCT03088033). IASD has been developed to lessen left atrial pressure by making an 8 mm hole in atrial septum so that blood goes through to right atrium. This trial is focused on HFpEF patients, since there has been no established pharmacological evidence for them. REDUCE LAP-HF I trial [14] showed that efficient decreases in pulmonary wedge pressure during exercise in the device group. Now phase III trial is going underway also in Japan.

References

1. Tsutsui H, et al. JCS 2017/JHFS 2017 guideline on diagnosis and treatment of acute and chronic heart failure- digest version. Circ J. 2019;83(10):2084–184.
2. Kinugawa K, Sato N, Inomata T. Effects of Tolvaptan on volume overload in patients with heart failure. Int Heart J. 2018;59(6):1368–77.
3. Imamura T, Kinugawa K. Update of acute and long-term Tolvaptan therapy. J Cardiol. 2019;73(2):102–7.
4. O'Connor CM, et al. Effect of nesiritide in patients with acute decompensated heart failure. N Engl J Med. 2011;365(1):32–43.
5. Metra M, et al. Effects of Serelaxin in patients with acute heart failure. N Engl J Med. 2019;381(8):716–26.
6. Van Gelder IC, et al. Lenient versus strict rate control in patients with atrial fibrillation. N Engl J Med. 2010;362(15):1363–73.
7. Nagai R, et al. Urgent management of rapid heart rate in patients with atrial fibrillation/flutter and left ventricular dysfunction: comparison of the ultra-short-acting beta1-selective blocker landiolol with digoxin (J-land study). Circ J. 2013;77(4):908–16.
8. Zelniker TA, et al. SGLT2 inhibitors for primary and secondary prevention of cardiovascular and renal outcomes in type 2 diabetes: a systematic review and meta-analysis of cardiovascular outcome trials. Lancet. 2019;393(10166):31–9.
9. McMurray JJV, et al. Dapagliflozin in patients with heart failure and reduced ejection fraction. N Engl J Med. 2019;381(21):1995–2008.
10. Armstrong PW, et al. Vericiguat in patients with heart failure and reduced ejection fraction. N Engl J Med. 2020; https://doi.org/10.1056/NEJMoa1915928. [Epub ahead of print].
11. Packer M, et al. Effect of oral milrinone on mortality in severe chronic heart failure. The PROMISE study research group. N Engl J Med. 1991;325(21):1468–75.
12. Marrouche NF, et al. Catheter ablation for atrial fibrillation with heart failure. N Engl J Med. 2018;378(5):417–27.
13. Mack MJ, et al. Transcatheter aortic-valve replacement with a balloon-expandable valve in low-risk patients. N Engl J Med. 2019;380(18):1695–705.
14. Feldman T, et al. Transcatheter interatrial shunt device for the treatment of heart failure with preserved ejection fraction (REDUCE LAP-HF I [Reduce elevated left atrial pressure in patients with heart failure]): a phase 2, randomized, sham-controlled trial. Circulation. 2018;137(4):364–75.

Chapter 2
Device Monitoring

Teruhiko Imamura

Abstract Abnormal hemodynamics is associated with poor clinical outcomes in patients with heart failure. Given the invasiveness and unfeasibility of routine right heart catheterization, remote noninvasive methodologies to monitor hemodynamics are needed. The CardioMEMS™ device is a recently developed technology that enables remote monitoring of pulmonary artery pressures via an implanted sensor most often located in the distal left pulmonary artery. Along with CardioMEMS™, Remote dielectric system might also be another promising device which reports indirect surrogates of intracardiac fillings pressures. In patients with advanced heart failure who require left ventricular assist devices, noninvasive hemodynamic monitoring is sorely needed given increased procedural risks of invasive assessments. The HVAD flow waveform is a variable under active investigation which might also provide an estimation of filling pressures. The methodology would lead to the concept of smart pump, which can adjust device setting automatically by monitoring hemodynamics.

Keywords Hemodynamics · Right heart failure · Unloading

2.1 Introduction

The implication of hemodynamic measurements in the management of heart failure (HF) patients has been a topic of great debate over the last two decades. The role of hemodynamic-guided medical therapy was investigated in the Evaluation Study of Congestive HF and Pulmonary Artery Catheterization Effectiveness (ESCAPE) Trial [1], an unblinded randomized control study, in which right heart catheterization (RHC) guided therapy did not improve short-term outcomes in patients with acute decompensated heart failure (ADHF). The study led to a significant reduction in the use of RHC in patients presenting with ADHF, even in those out of the inclusion criteria of ESCAPE. However, a post-hoc analysis of the ESCAPE trial found that persistently elevated cardiac filling pressure at posttreatment strongly predicted

T. Imamura (✉)
The Second Department of Internal Medicine, University of Toyama, Toyama, Japan

K. Kinugawa, T. Imamura (eds.), *Update of Non-Pharmacological Therapy for Heart Failure*, https://doi.org/10.1007/978-981-15-4843-7_2

worse clinical outcomes. These findings underscore the importance of identifying high-risk hemodynamic profiles in patients following attempted medical optimization.

There are several limitations in RHC-guided therapy for the treatment of patients presenting with ADHF [2]. The inherent primary risk lies in the invasiveness of the procedure and associated complications which can occur including infection, bleeding, and inadvertent arterial puncture. Second, continuous monitoring of hemodynamics in the inpatient setting is challenging and costly, requiring a stay in the intensive-care unit. Furthermore, static measures of hemodynamics through single evaluations may not always be the optimal strategy when managing clinically tenuous patients. In patients with severe structural heart disease, hemodynamic congestion might precede clinical congestion which often can be the precursor to triggering an admission for ADHF. Considering these limitations of traditional RHC and a high burden of disease-associated morbidity with HF, noninvasive remote devices to monitor hemodynamics are sorely needed. In this section, I will discuss several technologies that monitor hemodynamic parameters in both HF patients and those with left ventricular assist devices (LVAD).

2.2 Pulmonary Artery Pressure Monitoring (CardioMEMS™)

CardioMEMS is a recently debuted remote hemodynamic monitoring device [3], now increasingly used in both Europe and the United States. It is composed of a small sensor designed to be implanted in the main pulmonary artery via RHC, which then remotely monitors pulmonary artery pressures (PAP) (Fig. 2.1a). In 2014, CardioMEMS™ received approval from the Food and Drug Administration for the monitoring of PAP in patients with New York Heart Association Class III symptomology who have been hospitalized for HF [4]. CardioMEMS™ implantation also carries a class IIb recommendation from the European Society of Cardiology to monitor PAP in the symptomatic patients with HF with a previous HF hospitalization [5].

The CardioMEMS™ device is most commonly placed in the left distal pulmonary artery percutaneously via an over-the-wire system following an RHC in the cardiac catheterization laboratory (Fig. 2.1b). After pressure calibration, a continuous PAP waveform can be visualized (Fig. 2.1c). Figure 2.2 shows an example of a remote PAP monitoring interface. In general, PAP is measured by the patient once a day in the supine position, over the external antenna that activates the implanted CardioMEMS™ sensor. Wirelessly delivered PAP measurements are most often checked once per week or more by clinicians, triggering data-driven adjustments in HF-specific therapies. As shown in Fig. 2.2 at point A, PAP began to trend up often without any HF symptoms, but the clinician here can proactively address this change

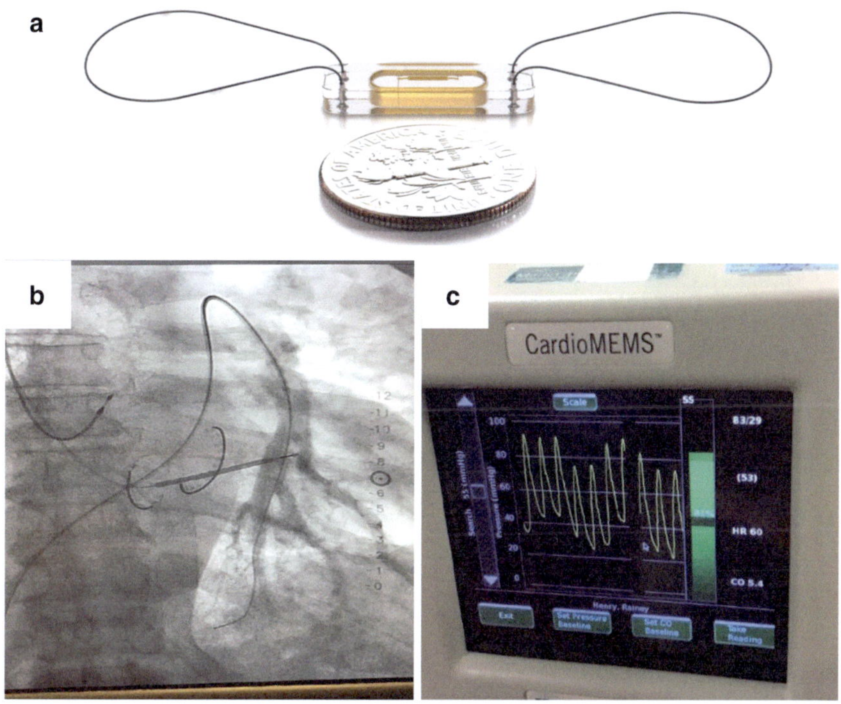

Fig. 2.1 CardioMEMS™ device (**a**) Angiography of left pulmonary artery to determine the optimal location of CardioMEMS™ implantation (**b**) Actual monitor of pulmonary artery pressures obtained from CardioMEMS™ located in the pulmonary artery (**c**)

by titrating the diuretic dose. At point B, PAP again increased despite adjustments in medical therapy, with the patient developing HF symptoms, triggering the clinician to hospitalization the patient for further assessment and treatment. The diastolic PAP is frequently used as a surrogate for pulmonary capillary wedge pressure (PCWP) except in scenarios of primary pulmonary arterial hypertension of out-of-proportion or "fixed" pulmonary hypertension due to left-HF.

Recently, in the CardioMEMS™ Heart Sensor Allows Monitoring of Pressure to Improve Outcomes in NYHA Class III HF Patients (CHAMPION) trial [6], use of CardioMEMS™ led to a 30% reduction in HF readmissions, equating to massive reductions in healthcare expenditures and reduced disease-specific morbidity. This outcome was probably attributed to a higher rate of changes to diuretic therapy and neurohormonal blockades in the group with active hemodynamic monitoring [7]. A larger GUIDE-HF trial is now underway recruiting 3600 patients to see if wider range of HF patients (NYHA II-IV) can have a HF-free survival benefit by CardioMEMS™ (Am Heart J. 2019 Aug;214:18-27. doi: https://doi.org/10.1016/j.ahj.2019.04.014. Epub 2019 May 3. Hemodynamic-GUIDEd management of Heart

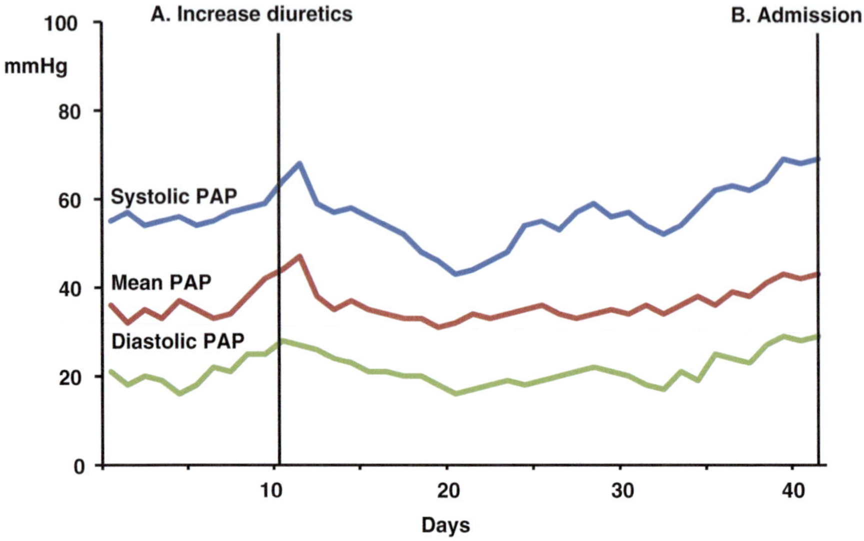

Fig. 2.2 An example of monitored pulmonary artery pressure interface in the CardioMEMS™ device

Failure (GUIDE-HF). Lindenfeld J [1], Abraham WT [2], Maisel A [3], Zile M [4], Smart F [5], Costanzo MR [6], Mehra MR [7], Ducharme A [8], Sears SF [9], Desai AS [7], Paul S [10], Sood P [11], Johnson N [11], Ginn G [11], Adamson PB [11]). Of note, this device has not yet been approved in Japan thus far.

2.3 Pulmonary Congestion Monitoring (Remote Dielectric System [ReDS])

ReDS employs low-power electromagnetic signals emitted between two sensors (one each on the anterior and posterior body surfaces) embedded in a wearable vest (Fig. 2.3a) [8]. The analyzed signal reflects the dielectric properties of the portion of the lung between the sensors. The dielectric coefficient of a material is represented by a frequency-dependent complex number describing its interaction with electromagnetic energy including the degrees of absorption, reflection, and transmission of the energy. Since water has a very high dielectric coefficient and air has a very low dielectric constant, the dielectric coefficient of a tissue is determined predominantly by its fluid content. This measurement takes 90 seconds to obtain.

Our team recently demonstrated that ReDS measurement correlated with actual PCWP by RHC (Fig. 2.3b) [9]. Given high sensitivity and moderate specificity, we suggest using ReDS technology for the screening of pulmonary congestion in the ambulatory setting. Intensive assessments including RHC should be considered when they have ReDS above 34% (cutoff to estimate PCWP >18 mmHg) to better risk-stratify patients and appropriately triage therapies. Further prospective trials

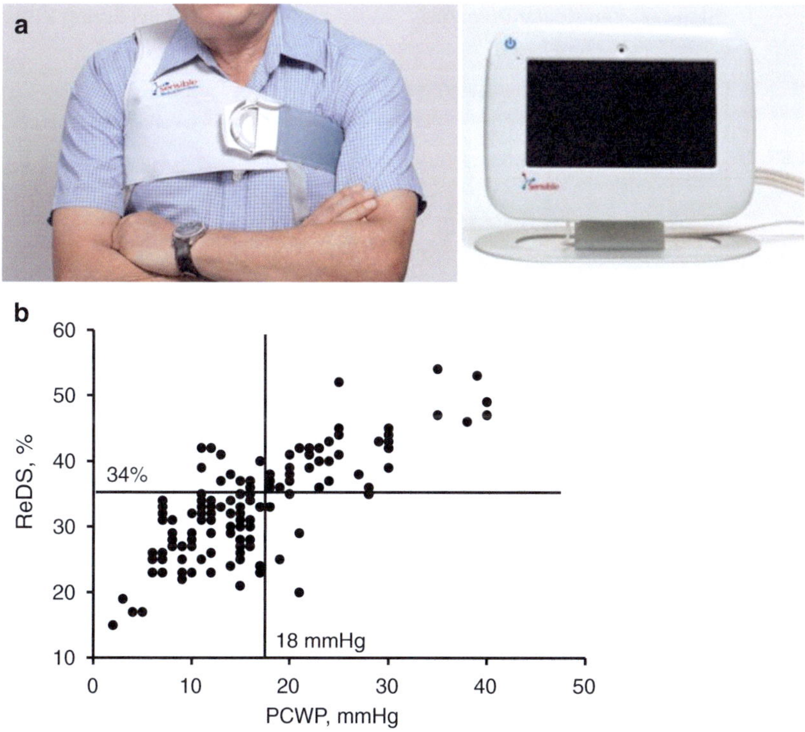

Fig. 2.3 Remote dielectric system (**a**) Correlation between actual measured pulmonary capillary wedge pressure and ReDS with each cutoff (**b**)

are needed to understand if ReDS-guided management improves in clinical outcomes in HF management [10].

2.4 Hemodynamic Monitoring in LVAD Patients

Hemodynamics measurements are also critically important in patients receiving LVAD support [2]. Recently, it has been demonstrated that hemodynamics are not necessarily optimized following LVAD implantation in a cohort of ambulatory, clinically stable patients [11]. Furthermore, abnormal hemodynamics in LVAD patients has been shown to be associated with worse clinical outcomes including HF readmissions and hemocompatibility-related adverse events [12]. Invasive hemodynamic optimization studies for LVAD patients combining simultaneous RHC and echocardiography to assess stepwise changes in filling pressures and ventricular size/valve opening (ramp test) may allow the clinician to choose a device speed that best suits the patient. Our team recently demonstrated in a prospective randomized control trial that patients who underwent hemodynamic ramp-guided management

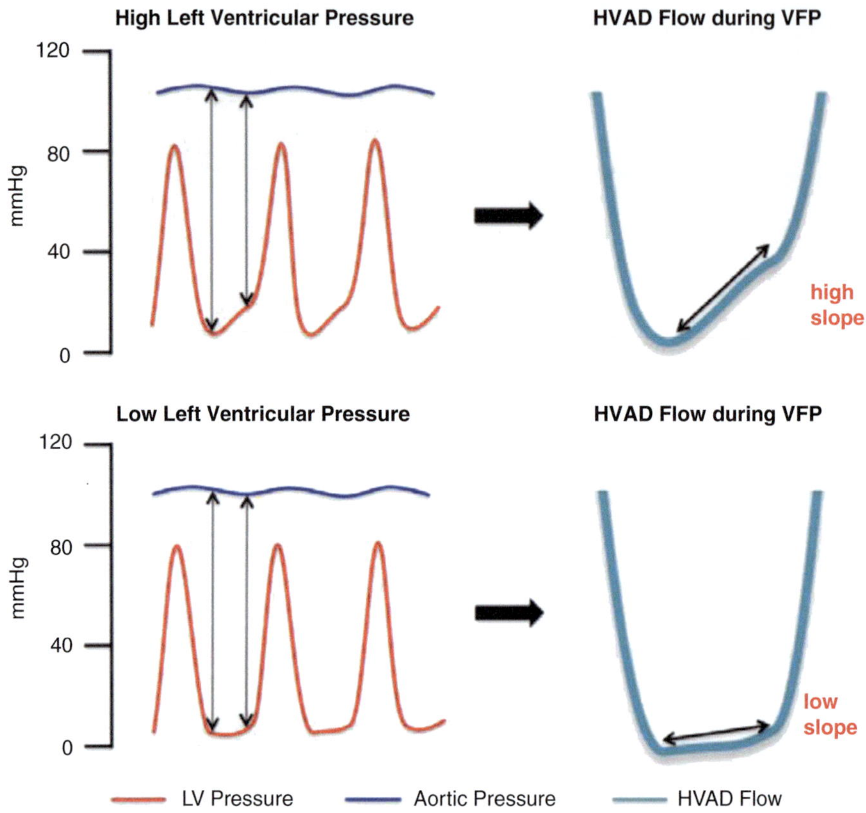

Fig. 2.4 Relationship between the actual left ventricular filling pressure (red line) and the diastolic slope of HVAD flow waveform. HVAD pump flow depends on the pressure gradient between left ventricle (red line) and aorta (blue line). When the pressure gradient drops, pump flow increases. Therefore, when left ventricular filling pressure increases in decompensated HF, the pressure gradient decreases and the diastolic slope of pump flow becomes increases. This is reused from [14] with permission

had reduced readmissions and more improved quality of life compared to the control group with conventional management (Ramp-it-Up trial) [13].

However, performing serial RHCs should be cautioned in LVAD patients given the increased risk of bleeding due to systemic anticoagulation. In lieu of this, non-invasive hemodynamic monitoring strategies are needed while managing patients with LVADs [2].

Recently, our team demonstrated that the slope of the flow waveform at the ventricular filling phase, which is displayed on the monitor of HVAD LVAD (Medtronic, Framingham, MA), had a strong correlation with actual measured PCWP (Fig. 2.4) [14]. Given how pump flow is dependent on the pressure gradient between the left ventricle and the aorta, elevations of left ventricular filling pressure seen in decompensated HF would reduce the pressure gradient in the pump resulting in increased flow. Based on this concept, we can estimate PCWP by measuring the slope of HVAD flow waveform at diastole.

In future smart pump designs which hope to automatically adjust flow based on the needs of the individual patient, machine-derived algorithms to assess the flow waveform slope and make appropriate device-speed changes will hopefully be present in next-generation devices. While it is not clear how far we are from the development of a smart pump, the understanding that the HVAD flow waveform provides valuable hemodynamic information is an important step forward.

Conflicts of Interest None.

References

1. Binanay C, Califf RM, Hasselblad V, O'Connor CM, Shah MR, Sopko G, Stevenson LW, Francis GS, Leier CV, Miller LW, Investigators E, Coordinators ES. Evaluation study of congestive heart failure and pulmonary artery catheterization effectiveness: the ESCAPE trial. JAMA. 2005;294(13):1625–33.
2. Imamura T, Chung B, Nguyen A, Sayer G, Uriel N. Clinical implications of hemodynamic assessment during left ventricular assist device therapy. J Cardiol. 2018;71(4):352–8.
3. Abraham WT, Adamson PB, Bourge RC, Aaron MF, Costanzo MR, Stevenson LW, Strickland W, Neelagaru S, Raval N, Krueger S, Weiner S, Shavelle D, Jeffries B, Yadav JS, Group CTS. Wireless pulmonary artery haemodynamic monitoring in chronic heart failure: a randomised controlled trial. Lancet. 2011;377(9766):658–66.
4. Loh JP, Barbash IM, Waksman R. Overview of the 2011 food and drug administration circulatory system devices panel of the medical devices advisory committee meeting on the CardioMEMS champion heart failure monitoring system. J Am Coll Cardiol. 2013;61(15):1571–6.
5. Ponikowski P, Voors AA, Anker SD, Bueno H, Cleland JGF, Coats AJS, Falk V, Gonzalez-Juanatey JR, Harjola VP, Jankowska EA, Jessup M, Linde C, Nihoyannopoulos P, Parissis JT, Pieske B, Riley JP, Rosano GMC, Ruilope LM, Ruschitzka F, Rutten FH, van der Meer P, Group ESCSD. 2016 ESC guidelines for the diagnosis and treatment of acute and chronic heart failure: the task force for the diagnosis and treatment of acute and chronic heart failure of the European Society of Cardiology (ESC) developed with the special contribution of the Heart Failure Association (HFA) of the ESC. Eur Heart J. 2016;37(27):2129–200.
6. Abraham WT, Stevenson LW, Bourge RC, Lindenfeld JA, Bauman JG, Adamson PB, Group CTS. Sustained efficacy of pulmonary artery pressure to guide adjustment of chronic heart failure therapy: complete follow-up results from the CHAMPION randomised trial. Lancet. 2016;387(10017):453–61.
7. Costanzo MR, Stevenson LW, Adamson PB, Desai AS, Heywood JT, Bourge RC, Bauman J, Abraham WT. Interventions linked to decreased heart failure hospitalizations during ambulatory pulmonary artery pressure monitoring. JACC Heart Fail. 2016;4(5):333–44.
8. Amir O, Azzam ZS, Gaspar T, Faranesh-Abboud S, Andria N, Burkhoff D, Abbo A, Abraham WT. Validation of remote dielectric sensing (ReDS) technology for quantification of lung fluid status: comparison to high resolution chest computed tomography in patients with and without acute heart failure. Int J Cardiol. 2016;221:841–6.
9. Uriel N, Sayer G, Imamura T, Rodgers D, Kim G, Raikhelkar J, Sarswat N, Kalantari S, Chung B, Nguyen A, Burkhoff D, Abbo A. Relationship between noninvasive assessment of lung fluid volume and invasively measured cardiac hemodynamics. J Am Heart Assoc. 2018;7(22):e009175.

10. Amir O, Ben-Gal T, Weinstein JM, Schliamser J, Burkhoff D, Abbo A, Abraham WT. Evaluation of remote dielectric sensing (ReDS) technology-guided therapy for decreasing heart failure rehospitalizations. Int J Cardiol. 2017;240:279–84.
11. Imamura T, Jeevanandam V, Kim G, Raikhelkar J, Sarswat N, Kalantari S, Smith B, Rodgers D, Besser S, Chung B, Nguyen A, Narang N, Ota T, Song T, Juricek C, Mehra M, Costanzo MR, Jorde UP, Burkhoff D, Sayer G, Uriel N. Optimal hemodynamics during left ventricular assist device support are associated with reduced readmission rates. Circ Heart Fail. 2019;12(2):e005094.
12. Imamura T, Nguyen A, Kim G, Raikhelkar J, Sarswat N, Kalantari S, Smith B, Juricek C, Rodgers D, Ota T, Song T, Jeevanandam V, Sayer G, Uriel N. Optimal haemodynamics during left ventricular assist device support are associated with reduced haemocompatibility-related adverse events. Eur J Heart Fail. 2019;21(5):655–62.
13. Uriel N, Burkhoff D, Rich JD, Drakos SG, Teuteberg JJ, Imamura T, Rodgers D, Raikhelkar J, Vorovich EE, Selzman CH, Kim G, Sayer G. Impact of hemodynamic ramp test-guided HVAD speed and medication adjustments on clinical outcomes. Circ Heart Fail. 2019;12(4):e006067.
14. Grinstein J, Rodgers D, Kalantari S, Sayer G, Kim GH, Sarswat N, Adatya S, Ota T, Jeevanandam V, Burkhoff D, Uriel N. HVAD waveform analysis as a noninvasive marker of pulmonary capillary wedge pressure: a first step toward the development of a smart left ventricular assist device pump. ASAIO J. 2018;64(1):10–5.

Chapter 3
CRT/ICD

Toshiko Nakai

Abstract Cardiac resynchronization therapy (CRT) is a standard therapy for patients with heart failure accompanied by conduction disturbance and dyssynchrony. However, we feel that this therapy is not sufficiently utilized, even 15 years after first being implemented. Acceptance level of this treatment differs among physicians and across regions, possibly due to the invasive nature of CRT, which has led to failure to introduce this treatment properly. However, indication of CRT should not be determined solely by the interest and opinion of the physician in charge. CRT is often indispensable in cases with conduction disturbance and impaired cardiac function, similar to the necessity for commencing beta-blocker treatment for heart failure. Failure to introduce this treatment is a deviation from standard therapy and requires a sufficient explanation for the reasons not selecting this treatment. The objective of this chapter is to confirm the indications for CRT and to share its efficacy, in the hope that this will serve as a guidance to appropriate treatment of heart failure, without delays in the introduction of CRT.

Keywords Cardiac resynchronization therapy · Heart failure · NHYA II · Intraventricular conduction disturbance · Cardiac dyssynchrony · Reverse remodeling

3.1 Introduction

We know that 10–30% of patients with advanced heart failure have intraventricular conduction disturbance [1–3]. In addition, patients with wide QRS have been observed to have a poorer prognosis than patients with normal QRS duration [4, 5]. CRT is a treatment developed for these circumstances [6], and the benefit of this treatment was confirmed by studying it in patients with dilated cardiomyopathy, a condition that was thought to be treatable by cardiac transplantation alone. The quality of life of these patients recovered dramatically, and they maintained their

T. Nakai (✉)
Department of Medicine, Division of Advanced Therapeutics for Cardiac Arrhythmias, Nihon University School of Medicine, Tokyo, Japan
e-mail: nakai.toshiko@nihon-u.ac.jp

K. Kinugawa, T. Imamura (eds.), *Update of Non-Pharmacological Therapy for Heart Failure*, https://doi.org/10.1007/978-981-15-4843-7_3

well-being for the rest of their lives. Many discoveries have been made in the 15-year history of CRT; however, there are many aspects which are still not well understood.

Patients with impaired cardiac function are known to have a high risk of sudden death due to fatal arrhythmias, and an implantable cardioverter defibrillator (ICD) is now used for primary prevention [7]. Therefore, many patients with an indication for CRT have a similar indication for a CRT defibrillator (CRT-D). However, in an aging Japanese society, there are many elderly patients with heart failure, which suggests that the additional risk of death due to arrhythmia may not be significant compared with the risk of death due to other causes. In addition, many of these patients are thought to be at risk of infection by implanting a thick, bulky ICD in a small body. For these reasons, CRT pacemakers (CRT-P) are selected in many cases.

Fifteen years have passed since the development of CRT, and although the efficacy of this treatment has been demonstrated, it has not at present been implemented widely enough. Percutaneous coronary intervention (PCI) is actively implemented in ischemic heart disease if stenosis is found in a coronary artery, so why is CRT not actively implemented in heart failure accompanied by a conduction disorder? Is there a margin for uncertainty in implementing CRT in patients who are repeatedly hospitalized for heart failure after administration of sufficient medication? It should be remembered that CRT is an essential treatment for patients with conduction disorders.

3.2 Indications for CRT

As suggested by many clinical studies conducted to date, patients who are expected to gain the greatest benefit from CRT are those with "complete left bundle branch block (CLBBB), QRS > 130 ms, NYHA functional class II, Sinus rhythm," and this is a class I recommendation, according to the guidelines. However, in clinical practice, there are many cases where CRT is considered effective despite not meeting these conditions. While the guidelines of the Japanese Circulation Society (JCS) recommend CRT for QRS > 120 ms [7], the ESC guidelines classify patients with QRS < 130 ms as "class III" that means they do not recommend this treatment [8]. The differences between these guidelines have had a significant effect on the introduction of CRT in Japanese patients, and many physicians seem to have difficulty deciding whether CRT should be introduced in patients with QRS < 130 ms and low cardiac function. According to the JCS guidelines, this group of patients has a class I indication and is expected to have a positive response to CRT.

The purpose of CRT is to improve the conduction disturbance. Drug treatment needs to be administered for the treatment of heart failure in order to reduce cardiac

Table 3.1 CRT recommendation. Modified from the JCS/JHFS guidelines

<table>
<tr><th></th><th>Class I</th><th>Class IIa</th><th>Class IIb</th><th>Class III</th></tr>
<tr><td rowspan="3">NYHA III/IV</td><td rowspan="3">① OMT
② LVEF ≤ 35%
③ LBBB, QRS ≥ 120 ms
④ SR</td><td>① OMT
② LVEF ≤ 35%
③ NLBBB,QRS ≥ 150 ms
④ SR</td><td rowspan="3">① OMT
② LVEF ≤ 35%
③ NLBBB,120 ≤ QRS ≤ 149 ms
④ SR</td><td rowspan="5">Patients whose physical function is limited by chronic conditions other than HF, or patients whose life expectancy is less than 12 months</td></tr>
<tr><td>①OMT
② LVEF<50%
③ PM/ICD indication
④ Expect V pacing</td></tr>
<tr><td>① OMT
② LVEF ≤ 35%
③ LBBB: QRS ≥ 120 ms, or, NLBBB: QRS ≥ 150 ms
④ Expect V pacing, Af</td></tr>
<tr><td>NYHA II</td><td>① OMT
② LVEF ≤ 30%
③ LBBB, QRS ≥ 150 ms
④ SR</td><td>① OMT
② LVEF ≤ 30%
③ NLBBB,QRS ≥ 150 ms
④ SR
② LVEF<50%
③ PM/ICD indication
④ Pacing dependent</td><td>① OMT
② LVEF ≤ 30%
③ NLBBB,120 ≤ QRS ≤ 149 ms
④ SR</td></tr>
<tr><td>NYHA I</td><td></td><td></td><td>① OMT
② LVEF < 50%
③ PM/ICD indication
④ Pacing dependent</td></tr>
</table>

Japanese Circulation Society/Japanese Heart Failure Society 2017. *OMT* optimal medical therapy, *LVEF* left ventricular ejection fraction, *(N) LBBB* (non) left bundle branch block, *SR* sinus rhythm, *PM* pacemaker, *ICD* implantable cardioverter/defibrillator, *Af* atrial fibrillation

work and for cardiac protection; however, conduction disturbances cannot be treated by medication. Even with current advances in medical treatment, pacing (electrical treatment) is the sole treatment available for conduction disturbances like sick sinus syndrome and atrioventricular block. Similarly, conduction disturbances such as CLBBB cannot be treated by medication. Conduction disturbances and dyssynchrony contribute to the further exacerbation of heart failure through persistent inefficiencies in cardiac contraction with every beat. CRT is a treatment that addresses this disorder. The recommendations for CRT in the JCS guidelines are shown in Table 3.1.

Case 1 demonstrates a patient who had a class I indication for CRT according to the JCS guidelines, despite a class III indication according to the ESC guidelines. This was an 80-year-old female with dilated cardiomyopathy who

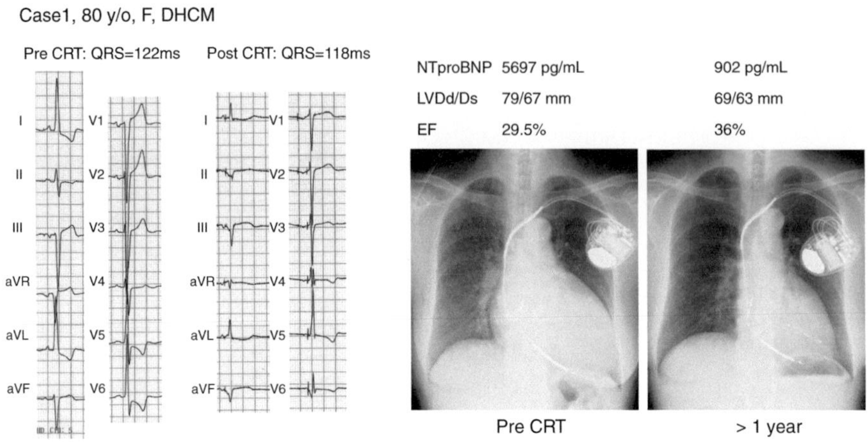

Fig. 3.1 An 80-year-old female patient. An implantable cardioverter defibrillator was implanted 7 years ago for dilated hypertrophic cardiomyopathy (DHCM) and ventricular tachycardia, and was upgraded to CRT-D due to gradual exacerbation of heart failure. The baseline electrocardiogram showed the QRS to be relatively narrow at 122 ms, and a narrow QRS was maintained after upgrading to CRT, with improvement in symptoms from NYHA III to NYHA I. *LVDd* left ventricular end-diastolic dimension, *Ds* end-systolic dimension, *EF* ejection fraction

responded to CRT (Fig. 3.1). The patient was elderly and not very active; however, her exercise tolerance was recovered, and her symptoms improved from NYHA III to NYHA I, allowing her to engage in activities such as housework and shopping.

3.3 CRT in Atrial Fibrillation

Unfortunately, CRT is not recommended as a class I indication in patients with atrial fibrillation (AF). CRT has been shown to exhibit a therapeutic effect by maintaining a high ventricular pacing rate, the patient thereby becoming a "responder" [9]. If spontaneous contraction is prioritized by an arrhythmia (such as AF) which results in the inhibition of ventricular pacing, the effect disappears instantly and tends to lower the response rate. For this reason, it is difficult to manage CRT in patients with AF, and some physicians determine that CRT is ineffective in patients with AF. Despite difficulties in management, sufficient efficacy can be expected if the pacing rate is maintained, and some of my own patients have even been "super-responders" (Fig. 3.2). Case 2 was a 61-year-old male patient with dilated cardiomyopathy (DCM) complicated by atrial fibrillation. Following the introduction of CRT in the context of NHYA class III heart failure, his symptoms improved markedly. His QRS has shortened (174 -> 120 ms) and cardiac function improved to a normal level of EF = 64%. He had been all-paced with CRT thanks to the high dose of beta-blocker administration as well as rate-response function of the device setting. This patient was an example of what is known as a "super responder."

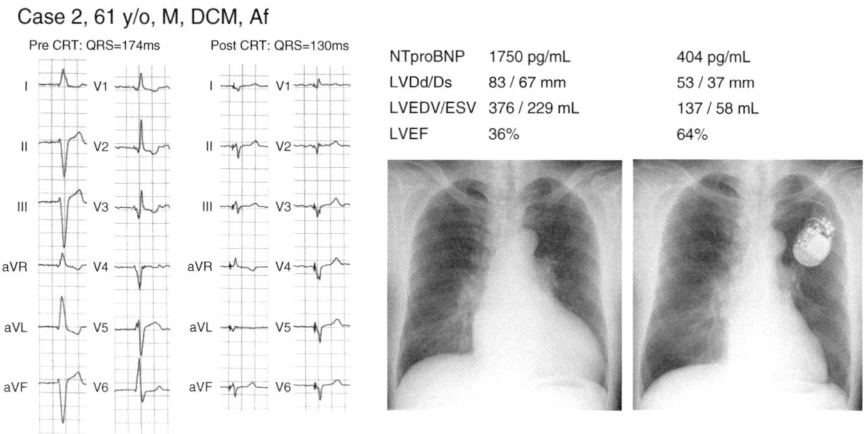

Fig. 3.2 A 61-year-old male patient with dilated cardiomyopathy (DCM) complicated by atrial fibrillation. The patient has impaired cardiac function and heart failure with NYHA functional class III, with a wide QRS accompanied by bifascicular block on electrocardiography, leading to the implantation of CRT-D according to the guidelines of the Japanese Circulation Society. Following the introduction of CRT, QRS was shortened to 120 ms and LVEF improved to 64%, with marked improvement in symptoms. *LVDd*, left ventricular end-diastolic dimension, *Ds* end-systolic dimension, *LVEDV* left ventricular end-diastolic volume, *Ds* end-systolic volume, *EF* ejection fraction

3.4 Timing of CRT Introduction

Figure 3.3 shows the course of heart failure. My experience in caring for patients with heart failure over time is supportive of the course of the disorder as shown in this figure. For the reasons shown in this figure, it is necessary that treatment be implemented as soon as possible to stop the progression of the disorder, and to achieve this, it is important to introduce available treatments as soon as possible. Although the indications for a left ventricular assist device (LVAD) and cardiac transplantation are shown in the JCS guidelines [10, 11], these are only applicable in patients with advanced heart failure who are at high risk of death. In addition, it is clear that these treatments are not easily accessible considering the circumstances regarding cardiac transplantation in Japan. Treatment must be applied to the fullest extent possible before the condition becomes too severe to avoid the necessity for an LVAD and cardiac transplantation. CRT is indicated for patients with a conduction disorder, even if the severity is mild or moderate (NYHA I and II). In fact, a poor prognosis has been reported with the introduction of CRT in the patients with advanced heart failure, and as a result, introduction at an early stage has been recommended [12]. In some cases, the QRS gradually becomes wider as heart failure progresses; therefore, regular examination of electrocardiography is recommended. Introduction of CRT at Stage D is considered too late; it is important to identify this indication during earlier stages, and avoid missing the timing of introduction so that treatment can be commenced by Stage C at the latest.

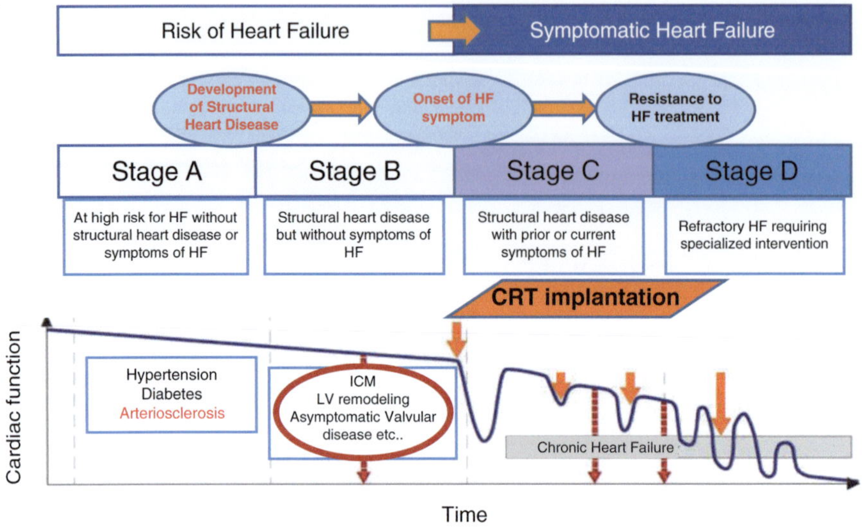

Fig. 3.3 Stages of heart failure. Modified from the JCS/JHFS Guidelines (2017)

3.5 CRT Programming

Compared with devices used in the initial stages of CRT treatment, these devices have undergone remarkable advances, enabling them to be programmed effectively for individual cases. QRS narrowing, which is an indication of conduction disturbance on the electrocardiogram, can be achieved easily using the algorithms installed on currently used devices, and this has led to an increase in the number of responders [13, 14]. However, these algorithms may not be compatible, depending on the implantation site of the right ventricular lead, the pattern of conduction disturbance, or the latency of the heart muscle; in such cases, a narrow QRS may not be achieved. When configuring the device at implantation or at outpatient visits, electrocardiography must be performed not only to check the QRS width but to determine the deviation in the timing of contraction between right and left ventricles, and AV delay and VV delay must be adjusted manually if necessary.

3.6 Attempts to Address Nonresponders

CRT is not only effective for improving dyssynchrony, but has also elicited a positive response in other cases, for example, those who were able to maintain their heart rate following implantation of CRT, leading to an increase in beta-blocker dosage; those in whom the signs of heart failure were detected by remote monitoring of CRT, thus preventing hospitalization due to heart failure; and those with improved insight into the disorder after implantation of CRT, leading to improvement in compliance with lifestyle guidance and medication. However, it should be kept in mind that CRT treatment is only an option in the treatment of heart failure (correcting dyssynchrony) and that the condition is not resolved (improved) merely by introducing CRT. There is a misconception that similar to the treatment of bradycardia, the implantation of CRT is thought to lead to recovery, possibly due to the nature of CRT as pacemaker treatment. However, this is a major misconception; heart failure cannot be resolved by CRT or medication alone, similar to the case where dilatation of coronary artery stenosis by PCI still requires additional treatments such as the suppression of arteriosclerosis, vasodilators, and lifestyle guidance.

Although the device itself has become more advanced and implantation techniques have improved, this does not prevent the occurrence of nonresponders. It has been reported that patients with advanced heart failure and patients with complications such as atrial fibrillation with insufficient maintenance of CRT pacing rate and frequent premature ventricular contraction (PVC) are likely to become nonresponders [15, 16]. Cases with advanced heart failure are difficult to manage; however, the most important measure is to use non-pharmacological treatments other than CRT to stabilize hemodynamics until efficacy with CRT is obtained, and most important of all to introduce CRT at an appropriate time before the condition becomes severe. For patients unable to maintain their CRT pacing rate due to arrhythmia, active measures should be taken, even considering implementation of AF ablation, PVC ablation, or AV node ablation [17, 18].

3.7 The Future of CRT

CRT was originally a means to correct conduction disturbance and dyssynchrony, and therefore provides an approach to aspects of heart failure that cannot be addressed by medication. It is expected that as more experience with CRT use is gained in Japan and the ways in which it can be used effectively are further explored, this will lead to the establishment of evidence that will allow CRT to be introduced simultaneously with beta-blockers, not just in moderate and more advanced heart failure, but also in mild cases with the initial diagnosis of heart failure.

References

1. Schoeller R, Andresen D, Buttner P, et al. First- or second-degree atrioventricular block as a risk factor in idiopathic dilated cardiomyopathy. Am J Cardiol. 1993;71:720–6.
2. Shenkman HJ, Pampati V, Khandelwal AK, McKinnon J. Congestive heart failure and QRS duration∗ establishing prognosis study. Chest. 2002;122:528–34.
3. Farwell D, Patel NR, Hall A, Ralph S, Sulke AN. How many people with heart failure are appropriate for biventricular resynchronization? Eur Heart J. 2000;21:1246–50.

4. Unverferth DV, Magorien RD, Moeschberger ML, Baker PB, Fetters JK, Leier CV. Factors influencing the one-year mortality of dilated cardiomyopathy. Am J Cardiol. 1984;54:147–52.
5. Shamim W, Francis DP, Yousufuddin M, et al. Intraventricular conduction delay: a prognostic marker in chronic heart failure. Int J Cardiol. 1999;70:171–8.
6. Abraham WT, Fisher WG, Smith AL, et al. Cardiac resynchronization in chronic heart failure. N Engl J Med. 2002;346:1845–53.
7. Guidelines for diagnosis and treatment of acute and chronic heart failure (JCS 2017/JHFS 2017). http://www.j-circ.or.jp/guideline/pdf/JCS2017_tsutsui_h.pdf
8. Ponikowski P, Voors AA, Anker SD, et al. European guidelines for the diagnosis and treatment of acute and chronic heart failure: the task force for the diagnosis and treatment of acute and chronic heart failure of the European Society of Cardiology (ESC) developed with the special contribution of the Heart Failure Association (HFA) of the ESC. Eur Heart J. 2016;37:2129–200.
9. Hayes DL, Boehmer JP, Day JD. Cardiac resynchronization therapy and the relationship of percent biventricular pacing to symptoms and survival. Heart Rhythm. 2011;8:1469–75.
10. Guidelines for device therapy: implantable left ventricular assist device for patients with severe heart failure (JCS/JSCVS 2013) http://www.j-circ.or.jp/guideline/pdf/JCS2013_kyo_h.pdf
11. Statement for heart transplantation (JCS 2016) http://www.j-circ.or.jp/guideline/pdf/JCS2016_isobe_h.pdf
12. Tang AS, Wells GA, Talajic M, et al. Cardiac-resynchronization therapy for mild-to-moderate heart failure. N Engl J Med. 2010;363:2385–95.
13. Filippatos G, Birnie D, Gold MR, et al. Rationale and design of the adapt response trial: a prospective randomized study of cardiac resynchronization therapy with preferential adaptive left ventricular-only pacing. Eur J Heart Fail. 2017;19:950–7.
14. Varma N, O'Donnell D, Bassiouny M, et al. Programming cardiac resynchronization therapy for electrical synchrony: reaching beyond left bundle branch block and left ventricular activation delay. J Am Heart Assoc. 2018;7:e007489.
15. Mullens W, Grimm RA, Verga T, Dresing T, Starling RC, Wilkoff BL, Tang WH. Insights from a cardiac resynchronization optimization clinic as part of a heart failure disease management program. Am Coll Cardiol. 2009;53:765–73.
16. Khatib M, Tolosana JM, Trucco E, et al. EAARN score, a predictive score for mortality in patients receiving cardiac resynchronization therapy based on pre-implantation risk factors. Eur J Heart Fail. 2014;16:802–9.
17. Lakkireddy D, Di Biase L, Ryschon K, et al. Radiofrequency ablation of premature ventricular ectopy improves the efficacy of cardiac resynchronization therapy in nonresponders. J Am Coll Cardiol. 2012;60:1531–9.
18. Gasparini M, Leclercq C, Lunati M, et al. Cardiac resynchronization therapy in patients with atrial fibrillation. The CERTIFY study (Cardiac resynchronization therapy in atrial fibrillation patients multinational registry). JAAC Heart Fail. 2013;1:500–7.

Chapter 4
Noninvasive Positive Pressure Ventilation

Shuji Joho

Abstract Although pharmacological therapy in heart failure is making rapid progress, the prevalence and mortality of heart failure remain high. Thus, effective non-pharmacological therapies combined with conventional therapies are essential for further improving the prognosis of heart failure. In recent years, noninvasive positive pressure ventilation (NPPV) therapy has been widely used for acute as well as chronic heart failure. This device, which is easy to wear and can be discontinued at any time, appears to have many advantages over other non-pharmacological therapies. Adaptive servo-ventilation (ASV) treatment has become common in clinical practice before large clinical trials have confirmed the prognostic superiority. Unfortunately, the large clinical trials of ASV have encountered unexpected negative results. However, could the evidence of small clinical studies cultivated so far be overwritten by large evidence? This review describes the role of NPPV therapy applied through a mask interface in the treatment of acute and chronic heart failure.

Keywords Noninvasive positive pressure ventilation · Continuous positive airway pressure · Adaptive servo-ventilation · Positive endo-expiratory pressure · Sleep disordered breathing · Obstructive sleep apnea · Central sleep apnea

4.1 Introduction

Noninvasive positive pressure ventilation (NPPV) is one of the non-pharmacological therapies in the treatment of chronic heart failure as well as acute heart failure. Continuous positive airway pressure (CPAP), bi-level positive airway pressure (BiPAP), Tri-level positive airway pressure, etc. have been used clinically and often show efficacy. First, we review the mechanisms of effectiveness of NPPV in the acute phase of heart failure. Second, we discuss CPAP and NPPV therapy for sleep disordered breathing with heart failure. Third, we focus on beneficial effects of adaptive servo-ventilation (ASV) for acute and chronic heart failure which

S. Joho (✉)
Second Department of Internal Medicine, University of Toyama, Toyama, Japan
e-mail: sjoho@med.u-toyama.ac.jp

K. Kinugawa, T. Imamura (eds.), *Update of Non-Pharmacological Therapy for Heart Failure*, https://doi.org/10.1007/978-981-15-4843-7_4

have been shown before 2015. Lastly, we mention about that the results of the multicenter randomized trial and show several concerns of the interpretation of the study results.

4.2 CPAP and NPPV (Including ASV) for Acute Pulmonary Edema and Acute Heart Failure, and the Mechanism of Effectiveness of Positive Pressure Treatment for Hemodynamics

In acute heart failure, when left atrial pressure is increased above 24 mmHg, fluid leakage into alveoli is also increased linearly, which results in pulmonary edema [1]. Nearly 90% of patients with acute heart failure have dyspnea, and most of them revealed lung congestion [2]. Importantly, dyspnea itself is the result of a complex interaction of physiological, environmental, and psychosocial factors [3]. In acute heart failure, dyspnea may be induced in four distinct settings: (1) increased ventilatory demand such as with hypoxic state, metabolic acidosis, or severe anemia; (2) decreased ventilatory capacity such as with pleural effusion, or muscle weakness; (3) increased airway resistance such as with asthma or chronic obstructive pulmonary disease; and (4) decreased pulmonary compliance such as with pulmonary edema [4]. However, less than 50% of patients present respiratory failure with hypoxemia because the mechanism of dyspnea is not simply via hypoxemia [5]. In acute heart failure, oxygen delivery capacity and tissue oxygen supply are reduced due to a decrease in cardiac output.

To date, the management has changed from ventilator management using endotracheal intubation to NPPV. In Japanese guidelines on acute heart failure, the early implementation of NPPV is recommended and is the first choice to reduce dyspnea in emergency ward [6]. Positive end-expiratory pressure (PEEP) improved breathing by preventing airway obstruction, reducing alveolar fluidity by improving alveolar collapse, reducing venous return, reducing pulmonary shunting, and reducing work of breathing [6]. Thus, in acute decompensated heart failure, application of NPPV is necessary to maintain oxygen saturation at a certain level or more to maintain tissue oxygenation. In addition, PEEP should reduce preload and afterload and which result in increase in cardiac output [7, 8]. PEEP acts as a sluice for venous return, acting on right ventricular (RV) unloading while increasing left ventricular end-diastolic volume through the interventricular septum and increasing stroke volume. The finding had been confirmed under both experimental and clinical settings [9, 10]. On the other hand, we should be careful that PEEP may be also detrimental because the increase in RV afterload may precipitate or aggravate RV failure [11].

For acute cardiogenic pulmonary edema, randomized trials revealed that CPAP improved respiratory failure faster than conventional oxygen therapy [12, 13] in

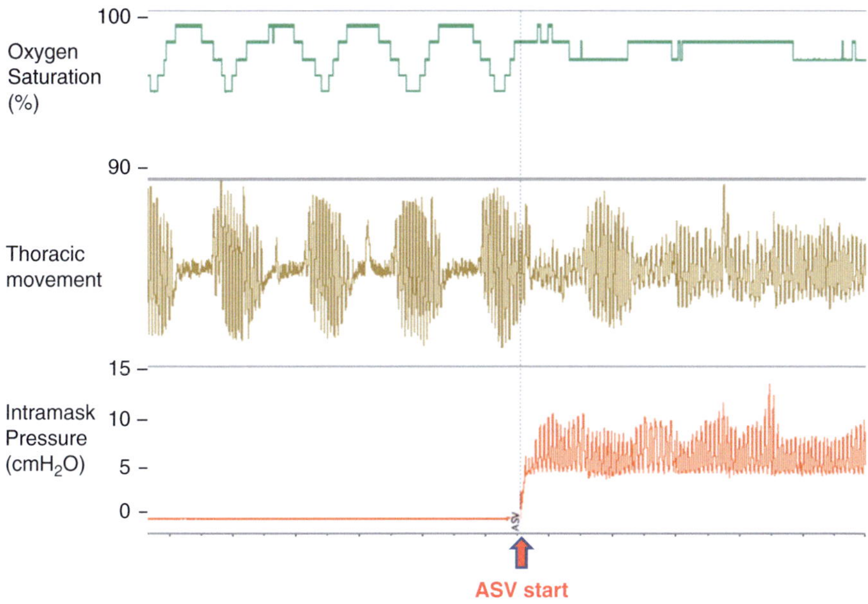

Fig. 4.1 Oxygen saturation level, respiratory pattern, and intramask pressure in a representative patient with heart failure and periodic breathing. Periodic breathing was apparent before, but was almost abolished during adaptive servo-ventilation

accompany with decreased endotracheal intubation rate. BiPAP also reached similar results in a randomized study [14]. Recent large randomized trial, including 1069 patients with acute cardiogenic pulmonary edema and respiratory acidosis, revealed that NPPV could improve respiratory distress faster than oxygen therapy; however, there was no difference in mortality between NPPV and conventional oxygen therapy. Because faster relief of dyspnea and respiratory distress is early goal of initial approach in patients with acute heart failure, NPPV should be selected as possible in the setting.

ASV is a method of ventilatory support designed for Cheyne–Stokes respiration (CSR). ASV can eliminate CSR as shown in Fig. 4.1. In Japan, ASV can be used in similar to CPAP and BiPAP in patients with acute decompensated heart failure under the support of the National Health Insurance. ASV could relieve dyspnea and improve hemodynamic status than standard oxygen alone [15, 16]. Additionally, it reduced the periods of intensive care unit stay and the hospitalization in comparison with conventional therapy [16]. ASV could also stop neurohumoral storm as shown by decrease in noradrenaline level [15]. However, it remains unclear whether ASV is truly superior to CPAP in the acute settings. The superiority of ASV over CPAP should be clarified in the acute setting.

4.3 CPAP and NPPV for Sleep Apnea Associated with Heart Failure and the Mechanism of Effectiveness of Positive Pressure Treatment for Apnea

Sleep disordered breathing is the most common comorbidity of heart failure. Up to 50% of patients have it; 21–40% exhibit central sleep apnea (CSA) or CSR, and 11–32% have obstructive sleep apnea (OSA) [17–20]. OSA is a risk factor for cardiovascular morbidity and mortality in the general population and deleterious to the cardiovascular system through mechanical, chemical, neurohumoral, and inflammatory mechanisms [21]. Intermittent hypoxia and hemodynamic changes along with sleep disturbance and sleep fragmentation are common in patients with OSA. These problems are important trigger for contributing to both the development of heart failure and the further precipitating of failing heart [22]. On the other hand, CSA with CSR likely occurs secondarily to the heart failure itself [23]. In CSA with CSR, intermittent hypoxia and hemodynamic changes along with sleep fragmentation, are also observed. Thus, sleep disordered breathing itself seemed important treatment target to relieve above detrimental mechanism of heart failure.

Recent guidelines in Japan recommended that OSA should be treated by CPAP in patients with heart failure (class I, level A) [6]. In randomized trial and meta-analyses of CPAP in patients with heart failure, CPAP improved left ventricular ejection fraction [24, 25]. Two observational study also revealed that CPAP improved their prognosis [26, 27]. The mechanism of the beneficial effect of CPAP is possibly via reduction of sympathetic activity, blood pressure, and the Epworth sleepiness scale, which might result in improvement of left ventricular ejection fraction.

Importantly, recent large scale clinical study (Sleep Apnea cardioVascular Endpoints: SAVE) had shown that use of CPAP had no significant effect on the prevention of recurrent serious cardiovascular events, despite significantly reduced sleepiness in patients with moderate to severe OSA and established cardiovascular disease (229 patients [17.0%] in the CPAP group vs. 207 patients [15.4%] in the normal care group: hazard ratio [HR] 1.10; 95% CI 0.91 to 1.32, $p = 0.34$) [28]. Insufficient daily use of CPAP (3.3 h/day) and inclusion of less severe OSA (moderate sleep apnea: apnea hypopnea index 15–30 events/h) might be attributable to the neutral results. However, in the subgroup analysis, the results of the propensity score matching analysis of 561 patients with good adherence and 561 patients in the normal care group showed that the events rate were also similar (15.3% vs. 17.5%, $p = 0.13$). Contrary to expectations, the group with higher oxygen desaturation index (> 30/h) for major combined outcomes did not show significant benefit. Additionally, patients with lower oxygen desaturation index tended to be more effective with CPAP. Although CPAP may be recommended for improving quality of life in symptomatic OSA patients, further investigation might be needed for indications of CPAP in patients with cardiovascular disease, especially heart failure.

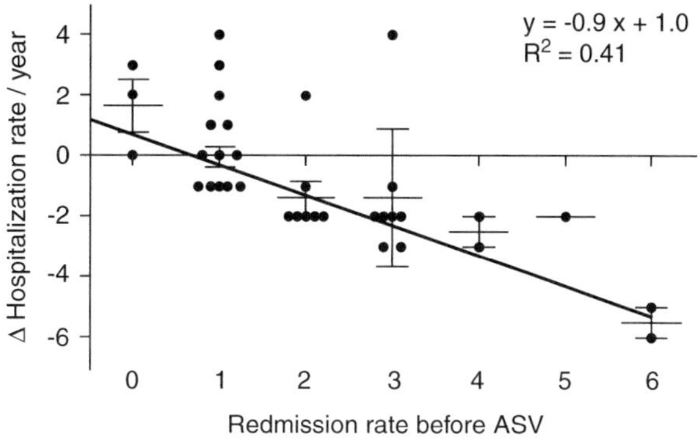

Fig. 4.2 The decrease tended to be greater in those patients with more frequent hospitalizations before ASV initiation (From reference [33])

4.4 Beneficial Effect of ASV Therapy for Chronic Heart Failure

In chronic heart failure, ASV also improves hemodynamics and symptoms of heart failure independent of improvement of sleep disordered breathing. Several observational studies indicated that ASV reduced cardiovascular outcomes in patients with heart failure irrespective of sleep disordered breathing [29–31]. Consistently, multicenter, randomized controlled trial (SAVIOR-C) also revealed that ASV could significantly reduce clinical composite endpoint in patients with heart failure [32]. ASV also reduced hospitalization frequencies from 1.9 ± 1.4 admissions in the 12 months before ASV to 1.1 ± 1.6 admissions in the 12 months after ASV initiation [33]. Importantly, the decrease tended to be greater in those patients with more frequent hospitalizations before ASV initiation (Fig. 4.2).

The mechanisms of the beneficial effect are via: (1) reducing pulmonary congestion, (2) reducing left ventricular preload and afterload, and (3) reducing sympathetic hyperactivity [6]. ASV exerted sympatholytic effects in patients with heart failure through inspiratory pressure support [34, 35] (Fig. 4.3). For example, inspiratory pressure support of BiPAP could decrease systemic and pulmonary vascular resistance, which might increase cardiac output via unloading of left and right ventricular afterload [36]. In contrast, the hemodynamic advantage of ASV over CPAP is not always observed in patients with heart failure: The higher the pulmonary capillary wedge pressure, the greater the difference in stroke volume between ASV and CPAP [37]. In experimental setting, acute increase of left atrial pressure directly contributed to breathing instability [38] (Fig. 4.4). Multicenter observational study had reported that respiratory instability increased as heart failure was deteriorated [39]. These findings suggest that the higher the intracardiac pressure, the greater the respiratory instability, which is the target of servo-ventilation, and the stronger the sympatholytic effect of ASV may be.

ASV was shown to not only improve exercise tolerance but also reduce periodic breathing during exercise [40, 41]. Changes in periodic respiration during exercise were significantly correlated with the degree of noradrenaline suppression, suggesting the beneficial effect of ASV on sympathetic nerve activity and CO_2 chemoreceptor sensitivity [41].

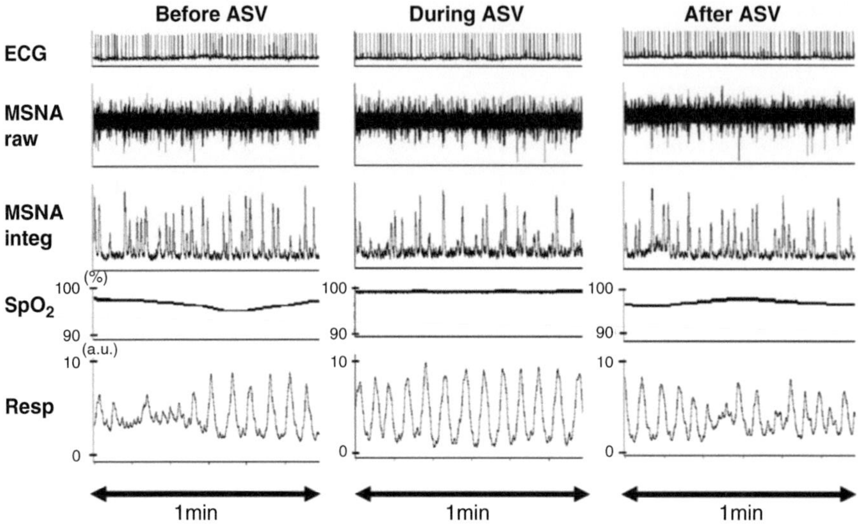

Fig. 4.3 Electrocardiograms (ECG), original and integrated signals of muscle sympathetic nerve activity (MSNA), oxygen saturation level (SpO_2), and respiratory pattern (Resp) in a representative patient with heart failure and periodic breathing (From reference [34]). Periodic breathing was apparent before (before ASV), but was almost abolished during adaptive servo-ventilation (during ASV). In this patient, MSNA decreased even after stopping ASV (after ASV)

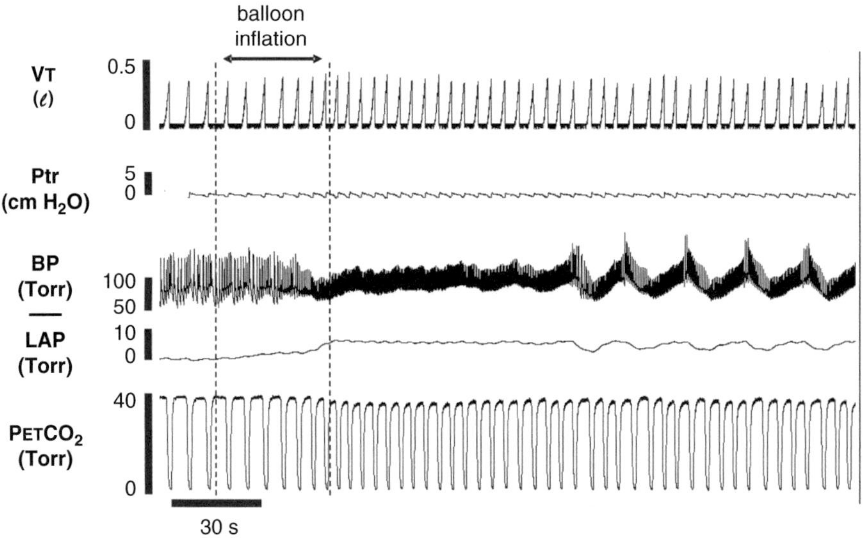

Fig. 4.4 Polygraph recording illustrating the spontaneous development of waxing and waning eupneic tidal volume (Vt), breathing frequency and blood pressure (BP) in response to increase of left atrial pressure (LAP) during balloon inflation which was located in left atrium (From reference [38]). The level of endo-tidal CO_2 ($EtCO_2$) was decreased during increase of LAP

4.5 Is ASV Therapy Really Harmful? Beyond the SERVE-HF Study

Although favorable reports of ASV in heart failure patients were continued before 2015, a large scale clinical study (Treatment of Sleep-Disordered Breathing With Predominant Central Sleep Apnea by Adaptive Servo-Ventilation in Patients With Heart Failure: SERVE-HF) warned about an increased risk of cardiovascular death associated with ASV for patients with CSA and chronic heart failure with reduced ejection fraction [42]. It was surprisingly inconsistent with earlier smaller studies and the negative results had a great impact on subsequent treatment guidelines [6]. The authors of the study explained the mechanisms of the increase in cardiovascular mortality as that CSA may be a compensatory mechanism in patients with heart failure, as has been suggested previously [43]. They suggested that the benefit of CSA and Cheyne–Stokes respiration could have been attenuated by ASV, and resulted in detrimental effect on heart failure. In fact, their subgroup analysis revealed that a positive association between the proportion of Cheyne–Stokes respiration and the adverse effect of ASV on cardiovascular mortality [42].

However, two previous reports might support the concept that their hypotheses cannot fully explain the unexpected results. The Canadian Continuous Positive Airway Pressure for Patients with Central Sleep Apnea and Heart Failure Trial: CANPAP, was a study comparing the efficacy of CPAP with a control group in heart failure patients with CSA who had reduced left ventricular ejection fraction [44]. In CANPAP study, CPAP resulted in a neutral result, but in the results of the sub-analysis, the prognosis was improved in the group in which apnea was decreased by CPAP at baseline (CPAP responder group), whereas the group in which apnea was not decreased (CPAP nonresponder group) did not improve the prognosis [45]. This result is one of the evidences to deny that suppressing CSA leads to worse prognosis. The other is a report by Kasai et al. They compared change in left ventricular ejection fraction between the group with continued CPAP versus the group with switching from CPAP to ASV because of CPAP nonresponder [46]. The left ventricular function was improved in the ASV group, but it was unchanged in the CPAP group. Consistently, in a non-randomized study, ASV improved left ventricular ejection fraction in association with suppression of CSA in patients with heart failure [47]. These facts that ASV effectively removed CSA and improved left ventricular ejection fraction are clearly different from the fact observed in this large trial.

Thus, we should further discuss why the ASV was detrimental in the SERVE-HF study, and why it was not detrimental in the earlier small reports. Several concerns were pointed out from the SERVE-HF study included over-pressurization and excessive crossover. The study protocol instructed manually increase of the expiratory and inspiratory positive airway pressures from the default levels to suppress sleep apnea. However, the effects of positive airway pressure on cardiac output depend on the baseline pulmonary-capillary wedge pressure [48]. Under euvolemic or hypovolemic status, application of positive pressure can deteriorate hemodynamics, which might result in increased cardiovascular death. Although ASV may be effective in some cases with heart failure with reduced ejection fraction, it is unclear which cases or which settings are truly beneficial for patients with heart failure. Therefore, it is appropriate not to use ASV for every case because of avoiding further harmful outcome. The SERVE-HF trial did not include heart failure with preserved ejection fraction, and the CAT-HF trial had positive results with heart failure with preserved ejection fraction [49], suggesting that ASV may reduce heart failure exacerbation in heart failure patients with preserved ejection fraction [50]. Because there are no agents to improve outcome in heart failure patients with preserved ejection fraction, it would be interesting if it is true. Also, in Japan, clinical trials of ASV for heart failure patients who are repeatedly hospitalized are ongoing. The results of this study are awaited to determine whether ASV is effective for heart failure patients with poor prognosis.

4.6 Conclusion

The findings about NPPV for heart failure were reviewed in this chapter. There are no doubts that NPPV is an effective non-pharmacological therapy in acute setting. However, further accumulation and advance of knowledge in this area should be waited in chronic heart failure.

References

1. Guyton AC, Hall JE. Chapter 38: Pulmonary circulation; Pulmonary edema; Pleural fluid. In: Guyton AC, Hall JE, editors. Textbook of medical physiology. Philadelphia: WB Saunders; 1996. p. 491–9.
2. Mebazaa A, Pang PS, Tavares M, Collins SP, Storrow AB, Laribi S, et al. The impact of early standard therapy on dyspnoea in patients with acute heart failure: the URGENT-dyspnoea study. Eur Heart J. 2010;31:832–41. https://doi.org/10.1093/eurheartj/ehp458.
3. Nishino T. Dyspnoea: underlying mechanisms and treatment. Br J Anaesth. 2011;106:463–74. https://doi.org/10.1093/bja/aer040.
4. Mukerji V. Chapter 11: Dyspnea, orthopnea, and paroxysmal nocturnal dyspnea. In: Walker HK, Hall WD, Hurst JW, editors. Clinical methods: the history, physical, and laboratory examinations. 3rd ed. Boston, MA: Butterworths; 1990. p. 78–80.
5. Park JJ, Choi DJ, Yoon CH, Oh IY, Lee JH, Ahn S, et al. The prognostic value of arterial blood gas analysis in high-risk acute heart failure patients: an analysis of the Korean Heart Failure (KorHF) registry. Eur J Heart Fail. 2015;17:601–11. https://doi.org/10.1002/ejhf.276.
6. Tsutsui H, Isobe M, Ito H, Ito H, Okumura K, Ono M, et al. JCS 2017/JHFS 2017 guideline on diagnosis and treatment of acute and chronic heart failure – digest version. Circ J. 2019;83:2084–184. https://doi.org/10.1253/circj.CJ-19-0342.
7. Pinsky MR, Summer WR, Wise RA, Permutt S, Bromberger-Barnea B. Augmentation of cardiac function by elevation of intrathoracic pressure. J Appl Physiol Respir Environ Exerc Physiol. 1983;54:950–5.
8. Bradley TD, Holloway RM, McLaughlin PR, Ross BL, Walters J, Liu PP. Cardiac output response to continuous positive airway pressure in congestive heart failure. Am Rev Respir Dis. 1992 Feb;145(2 Pt 1):377–82.

9. Mitchell JR, Whitelaw WA, Sas R, Smith ER, Tyberg JV, Belenkie I. RV filling modulates LV function by direct ventricular interaction during mechanical ventilation. Am J Physiol Heart Circ Physiol. 2005;289:H549–57.
10. Imamura T, Kinugawa K. Right ventricular end-diastolic pressure is a key to the changes in cardiac output during adaptive servo-ventilation support in patients with heart failure. Int Heart J. 2017;58:536–43. https://doi.org/10.1536/ihj.16-489.
11. Harjola VP, Mebazaa A, Čelutkienė J, Bettex D, Bueno H, Chioncel O, et al. Contemporary management of acute right ventricular failure: a statement from the Heart Failure Association and the Working Group on Pulmonary Circulation and Right Ventricular Function of the European Society of Cardiology. Eur J Heart Fail. 2016;18:226–41. https://doi.org/10.1002/ejhf.478.
12. Räsänen J, Heikkilä J, Downs J, Nikki P, Väisänen I, Viitanen A. Continuous positive airway pressure by face mask in acute cardiogenic pulmonary edema. Am J Cardiol. 1985;55:296–300.
13. Bersten AD, Holt AW, Vedig AE, Skowronski GA, Baggoley CJ. Treatment of severe cardiogenic pulmonary edema with continuous positive airway pressure delivered by face mask. N Engl J Med. 1991;325:1825–30.
14. Masip J, Betbesé AJ, Páez J, Vecilla F, Cañizares R, Padró J, et al. Non-invasive pressure support ventilation versus conventional oxygen therapy in acute cardiogenic pulmonary oedema: a randomised trial. Lancet. 2000;356:2126–32.
15. Nakano S, Kasai T, Tanno J, Sugi K, Sekine Y, Muramatsu T, et al. The effect of adaptive servo-ventilation on dyspnoea, haemodynamic parameters and plasma catecholamine concentrations in acute cardiogenic pulmonary oedema. Eur Heart J Acute Cardiovasc Care. 2015;4:305–15. https://doi.org/10.1177/2048872614549103.
16. Kinoshita M, Okayama H, Kawamura G, Shigematsu T, Takahashi T, Kawata Y, et al. Beneficial effects of rapid introduction of adaptive servo-ventilation in the emergency room in patients with acute cardiogenic pulmonary edema. J Cardiol. 2017;69:308–13. https://doi.org/10.1016/j.jjcc.2016.05.015.
17. Javaheri S, Parker TJ, Liming JD, Corbett WS, Nishiyama H, Wexler L, et al. Sleep apnea in 81 ambulatory male patients with stable heart failure. Types and their prevalences, consequences, and presentations. Circulation. 1998;97:2154–9.
18. Sin DD, Fitzgerald F, Parker JD, Newton G, Floras JS, Bradley TD. Risk factors for central and obstructive sleep apnea in 450 men and women with congestive heart failure. Am J Respir Crit Care Med. 1999;160:1101–6.
19. Vazir A, Hastings PC, Dayer M, McIntyre HF, Henein MY, Poole-Wilson PA, et al. A high prevalence of sleep disordered breathing in men with mild symptomatic chronic heart failure due to left ventricular systolic dysfunction. Eur J Heart Fail. 2007;9:243–50.
20. Yumino D, Wang H, Floras JS, Newton GE, Mak S, Ruttanaumpawan P, et al. Prevalence and physiological predictors of sleep apnea in patients with heart failure and systolic dysfunction. J Card Fail. 2009;15:279–85. https://doi.org/10.1016/j.cardfail.2008.11.015.
21. Bradley TD, Floras JS. Sleep apnea and heart failure: Part I: obstructive sleep apnea. Circulation. 2003;107:1671–8.
22. Dempsey JA, Veasey SC, Morgan BJ, O'Donnell CP. Pathophysiology of sleep apnea. Physiol Rev. 2010;90:47–112. https://doi.org/10.1152/physrev.00043.2008.
23. Yumino D, Bradley TD. Central sleep apnea and Cheyne-Stokes respiration. Proc Am Thorac Soc. 2008;5:226–36. https://doi.org/10.1513/pats.200708-129MG.
24. Kaneko Y, Floras JS, Usui K, Plante J, Tkacova R, Kubo T, et al. Cardiovascular effects of continuous positive airway pressure in patients with heart failure and obstructive sleep apnea. N Engl J Med. 2003;348:1233–41.
25. Mansfield DR, Gollogly NC, Kaye DM, Richardson M, Bergin P, Naughton MT. Controlled trial of continuous positive airway pressure in obstructive sleep apnea and heart failure. Am J Respir Crit Care Med. 2004;169:361–6.
26. Kasai T, Narui K, Dohi T, Yanagisawa N, Ishiwata S, Ohno M, et al. Prognosis of patients with heart failure and obstructive sleep apnea treated with continuous positive airway pressure. Chest. 2008;133:690–6. https://doi.org/10.1378/chest.07-1901.

27. Damy T, Margarit L, Noroc A, Bodez D, Guendouz S, Boyer L, et al. Prognostic impact of sleep-disordered breathing and its treatment with nocturnal ventilation for chronic heart failure. Eur J Heart Fail. 2012;14:1009–19. https://doi.org/10.1093/eurjhf/hfs085.
28. McEvoy RD, Antic NA, Heeley E, Luo Y, Ou Q, Zhang X, et al. CPAP for prevention of cardiovascular events in obstructive sleep apnea. N Engl J Med. 2016;375:919–31. https://doi.org/10.1056/NEJMoa1606599.
29. Koyama T, Watanabe H, Igarashi G, Terada S, Makabe S, Ito H. Short-term prognosis of adaptive servo-ventilation therapy in patients with heart failure. Circ J. 2011;75:710–2.
30. Takama N, Kurabayashi M. Effectiveness of adaptive servo-ventilation for treating heart failure regardless of the severity of sleep-disordered breathing. Circ J. 2011;75:1164–9.
31. Imamura T, Kinugawa K, Nitta D, Komuro I. Long-term adaptive servo-ventilator treatment prevents cardiac death and improves clinical outcome. Int Heart J. 2016;57:47–52. https://doi.org/10.1536/ihj.15-229.
32. Momomura S, Seino Y, Kihara Y, Adachi H, Yasumura Y, Yokoyama H, et al. Adaptive servo-ventilation therapy for patients with chronic heart failure in a confirmatory, multicenter, randomized, controlled study. Circ J. 2015;79:981–90. https://doi.org/10.1253/circj.CJ-15-0221.
33. Yoshida M, Ando SI, Kodama K, Ebihara K, Tanaka K, Hayashi A, et al. Adaptive servo-ventilation therapy reduces hospitalization rate in patients with severe heart failure. Int J Cardiol. 2017;238:173–6. https://doi.org/10.1016/j.ijcard.2017.02.075.
34. Harada D, Joho S, Oda Y, Hirai T, Asanoi H, Inoue H. Short term effect of adaptive servo-ventilation on muscle sympathetic nerve activity in patients with heart failure. Auton Neurosci. 2011;161:95–102. https://doi.org/10.1016/j.autneu.2010.12.001.
35. Ushijima R, Joho S, Akabane T, Oda Y, Inoue H. Differing effects of adaptive servoventilation and continuous positive airway pressure on muscle sympathetic nerve activity in patients with heart failure. Circ J. 2014;78:1387–95.
36. Yoshida M, Kadokami T, Momii H, Hayashi A, Urashi T, Narita S, et al. Enhancement of cardiac performance by bilevel positive airway pressure ventilation in heart failure. J Card Fail. 2012;18:912–8. https://doi.org/10.1016/j.cardfail.2012.10.009.
37. Asakawa N, Sakakibara M, Noguchi K, Kamiya K, Yamada S, Yoshitani T, et al. Adaptive servo-ventilation has more favorable acute effects on hemodynamics than continuous positive airway pressure in patients with heart failure. Int Heart J. 2015;56:527–32. https://doi.org/10.1536/ihj.15-110.
38. Chenuel BJ, Smith CA, Skatrud JB, Henderson KS, Dempsey JA. Increased propensity for apnea in response to acute elevations in left atrial pressure during sleep in the dog. J Appl Physiol (1985). 2006;101:76–83.
39. Takagawa J, Asanoi H, Tobushi T, Kumagai N, Kadokami T, Dohi K, et al. Multicenter, prospective study on respiratory stability during recovery from deterioration of chronic heart failure. Circ J. 2018;83:164–73. https://doi.org/10.1253/circj.CJ-18-0519.
40. Oldenburg O, Bitter T, Lehmann R, Korte S, Dimitriadis Z, Faber L, et al. Adaptive servoventilation improves cardiac function and respiratory stability. Clin Res Cardiol. 2011;100:107–15. https://doi.org/10.1007/s00392-010-0216-9.
41. Joho S, Ushijima R, Akabane T, Oda Y, Inoue H. Adaptive servo-ventilation improves exercise oscillatory ventilation and ventilatory inefficiency in patients with heart failure and central sleep apnea. IJC Metabolic & Endocrine. 2013;1:20–6. https://doi.org/10.1016/j.ijcme.2013.11.001.
42. Cowie MR, Woehrle H, Wegscheider K, Angermann C, d'Ortho MP, Erdmann E, et al. Adaptive servo-ventilation for central sleep apnea in systolic heart failure. N Engl J Med. 2015;373:1095–105. https://doi.org/10.1056/NEJMoa1506459.
43. Naughton MT. Cheyne-Stokes respiration: friend or foe? Thorax. 2012;67:357–60. https://doi.org/10.1136/thoraxjnl-2011-200927.
44. Bradley TD, Logan AG, Kimoff RJ, Sériès F, Morrison D, Ferguson K, et al. Continuous positive airway pressure for central sleep apnea and heart failure. N Engl J Med. 2005;353:2025–33.

45. Arzt M, Floras JS, Logan AG, Kimoff RJ, Series F, Morrison D, et al. Suppression of central sleep apnea by continuous positive airway pressure and transplant-free survival in heart failure: a post hoc analysis of the Canadian continuous positive airway pressure for patients with central sleep apnea and heart failure trial (CANPAP). Circulation. 2007;115:3173–80.
46. Kasai T, Kasagi S, Maeno K, Dohi T, Kawana F, Kato M, et al. Adaptive servo-ventilation in cardiac function and neurohormonal status in patients with heart failure and central sleep apnea nonresponsive to continuous positive airway pressure. JACC Heart Fail. 2013;1:58–63. https://doi.org/10.1016/j.jchf.2012.11.002.
47. Joho S, Oda Y, Ushijima R, Hirai T, Inoue H. Effect of adaptive servoventilation on muscle sympathetic nerve activity in patients with chronic heart failure and central sleep apnea. J Card Fail. 2012;18:769–75. https://doi.org/10.1016/j.cardfail.2012.08.360.
48. Kihara Y, Seino Y, Momomura S, SAVIOR-C investigators. Adaptive servo-ventilation for central sleep apnea in heart failure. N Engl J Med. 2016;374:687–8. https://doi.org/10.1056/NEJMc1515007.
49. O'Connor CM, Whellan DJ, Fiuzat M, Punjabi NM, Tasissa G, Anstrom KJ, et al. Cardiovascular outcomes with minute ventilation-targeted adaptive servo-ventilation therapy in heart failure: the CAT-HF trial. J Am Coll Cardiol. 2017;69:1577–87. https://doi.org/10.1016/j.jacc.2017.01.041.
50. Yoshihisa A, Suzuki S, Yamaki T, Sugimoto K, Kunii H, Nakazato K, et al. Impact of adaptive servo-ventilation on cardiovascular function and prognosis in heart failure patients with preserved left ventricular ejection fraction and sleep-disordered breathing. Eur J Heart Fail. 2013;15:543–50. https://doi.org/10.1093/eurjhf/hfs197.

Chapter 5
Comprehensive Cardiac Rehabilitation

Shintaro Kinugawa

Abstract Exercise tolerance declines in individuals with heart failure (HF), and this loss of exercise tolerance is an important indicator of the severity of HF and a predictor of prognosis. Exercise therapy including aerobic exercise and/or resistance exercise is necessary to improve and prevent this decline in exercise tolerance. Considering the pathology of HF, it is also necessary to establish a multidisciplinary disease management program for its treatment. In this chapter, the importance of exercise therapy and multidisciplinary disease management programs are outlined from the viewpoint of the pathophysiology of HF. The program that integrates these two is comprehensive cardiac rehabilitation itself. Comprehensive cardiac rehabilitation should be considered the standard treatment for HF alongside drug therapy. Medical staff involved in HF treatment must work on comprehensive cardiac rehabilitation.

Keywords Exercise capacity · Exercise therapy · Disease management program · Aerobic exercise · Resistance exercise · Sarcopenia · Anaerobic threshold

5.1 Treatments for HF

In the American Heart Association/American College of Cardiology (AHA/ACC) classification of the stages of HF, patients with asymptomatic HF who have structural heart disease are considered stage B. Patients with symptomatic HF and structural heart disease, including those with a history of HF, are stage C. Patients with refractory HF who have continued to be New York Heart Association (NYHA) functional class III or IV HF despite all available drug therapy or nonpharmacologic therapy with proven efficacy and are hospitalized for HF at least 2×/year are classified as stage D. This indicates that HF is a progressive disease condition.

Individuals with heart failure (HF) show various clinical symptoms due to organ congestion and peripheral hypoperfusion based on reduced cardiac pump

S. Kinugawa (✉)
Division of Cardiovascular Medicine, Research Institute of Angiocardiology, Graduate School of Medical Sciences, Kyushu University, Fukuoka, Japan
e-mail: kinugawa@cardiol.med.kyushu-u.ac.jp

K. Kinugawa, T. Imamura (eds.), *Update of Non-Pharmacological Therapy for Heart Failure*, https://doi.org/10.1007/978-981-15-4843-7_5

function. In the NYHA functional classification, the severity is classified according to symptoms that are observed in daily life, including exercise tolerance. There are various determinants of exercise tolerance, but it can be said that exercise tolerance is an index that reflects the severity of the condition of the whole body, considering the pathology of HF. Indeed, peak oxygen uptake is an independent prognostic factor.

HF is a progressive disease condition that leads to death with repeated exacerbations. In this process, the activation of neurohumoral factors is related to the development of myocardial remodeling [1], and the inhibition of this activation by drugs forms the basis of the treatment of HF. The most important treatment in HF is drug therapy. The inhibitors of neurohumoral factor that play an important role in the development of HF are widely used for patients with all severity levels of HF [2]. Diuretics are required if there is organ congestion. If the HF becomes more severe, treatment using various devices is performed. On other hand, exercise therapy and disease management programs apply to almost all patients with HF.

5.2 Effects of Exercise Therapy

It is established that properly prescribed exercise therapy can provide multifaceted benefits for HF patients. It is effective for the heart, coronary arteries, skeletal muscle, blood vessels, autonomic nerves, ventilation, inflammation, and more. These beneficial effects result in improvements of an individual's exercise capacity, quality of life (QOL), and long-term morality (Figs. 5.1 and 5.2). Exercise therapy increases the peak oxygen uptake by 15%–30% (average 20%) and improves the anaerobic threshold (AT). Such improvements in exercise capacity are due to an increase in skeletal muscle mass, an increase in skeletal muscle mitochondrial volume and function, a normalization of the fiber-type shift (i.e., a decrease in type I fibers and an increase in IIb fibers), and improvements in skeletal muscle energy metabolism and respiratory muscle function, and an improvement in vasodilator response through an increased expression of nitric oxide synthase.

Exercise therapy also combats chronic inflammation and autonomic nerve function (by suppressing sympathetic nerves and activating parasympathetic nerves), which play an important role in the progression of HF. These effects may be closely related to the improvement in mortality. In contrast, the effect of exercise therapy on cardiac function and myocardial remodeling is not great. Nevertheless, exercise therapy has beneficial effects on aspects of mental health such as anxiety and depression, leading to an improved QOL.

Many research groups have reported a beneficial effect of exercise therapy on the long-term prognosis of patients with HF. In their study of patients with chronic HF, Belardinelli et al. reported that compared to a non-exercise therapy group, the relative risk of cardiac death was reduced by 63% in the exercise therapy group [3]. The findings from the Exercise Training Meta-Analysis of Trials in Chronic Heart Failure (ExTraMATCH) revealed that exercise therapy improved the prognosis of

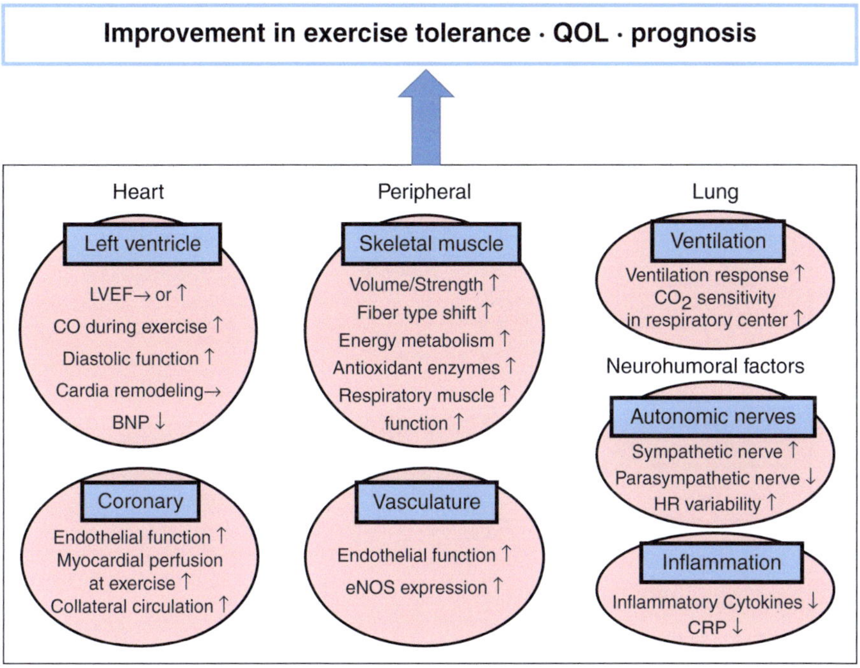

Fig. 5.1 Effects of exercise therapy. BNP: brain natriuretic peptide, *CO*, cardiac output, CO_2, carbon dioxide, *CRP*, C-reactive protein, *eNOS*, endothelial nitric oxide synthase, *HR*, heart rate, *LVEF*, left ventricular ejection fraction. ↑ indicates "increase," "improvement," or "normalization," → indicates "no change." ↓ indicates "decrease"

patients with HF [4]. The large-scale randomized trial HF-ACTION demonstrated safety and QOL improvements provided by exercise therapy in patients with chronic HF [5]. In that trial, exercise therapy also decreased the risk of all-cause death or hospitalization by 11% and the risk of cardiovascular death or hospitalization for HF by 15% after adjusting for confounding factors.

5.3 Exercise Prescription for HF

An exercise training program for a patient with HF consists of (1) a warm-up, (2) endurance exercise, (3) low-intensity resistance exercise, and (4) cooldown. At the stable phase of HF, it is recommended that patients perform a warm-up for 10–20 min, endurance exercise for 30–60 min, and cooldown for 5–10 min. Recommended endurance exercises are indoor walking, a cycle ergometer, and light aerobics. Jogging, swimming, and vigorous aerobic dance are not recommended because of the high risk of HF worsening due to the high load provided by these activities.

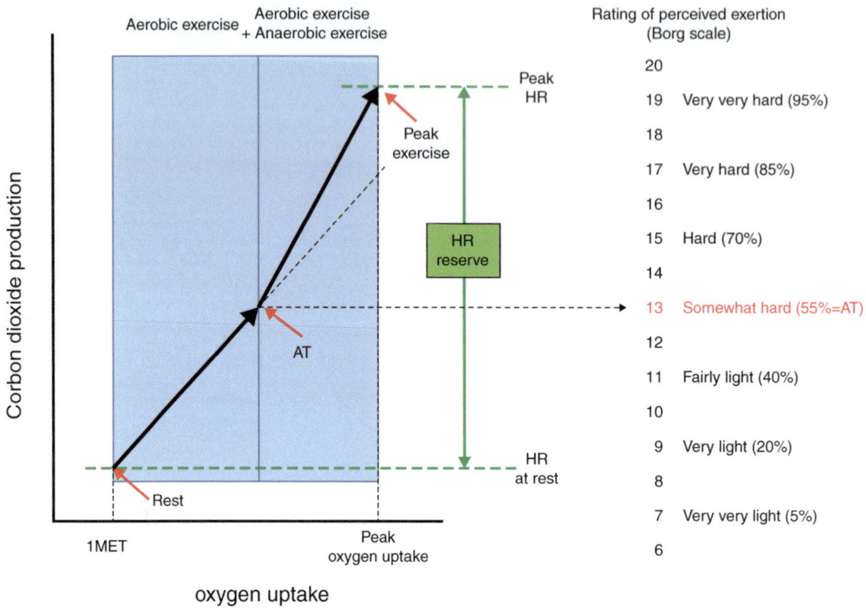

Fig. 5.2 Cardiopulmonary exercise test and Borg scale. *AT*, anaerobic threshold, *HR*, heart rate, *MET*, metabolic equivalent

At the beginning of exercise therapy, low-intensity exercise (indoor walking at 50–80 m/min for 5–10 min or a cycle ergometer at 10–20 W for 5–10 min) is started at 2×/day. The duration and intensity of exercise should be increased gradually over 1 month as guided by the patient's signs and symptoms during exercise. The selection of the exercise intensity should be based on the patient's resting heart rate + 30 beats/min (+20 beats/min for a patient using a β-blocker) as the target heart rate.

The most objective method of exercise prescription for patients at the stable phase of HF is a prescription based on the AT revealed by a cardiopulmonary exercise test. Essentially, with low-intensity exercise, the exercise program can be continued as only aerobic exercise, but when the exercise intensity is gradually increased, sufficient energy cannot be obtained with aerobic exercise alone, and anaerobic exercise is added. This point is called the AT (Fig. 5.2). The target heart rate is set at 40%–60% of the peak oxygen uptake or it is set at the AT. When the oxygen uptake could not be measured, the heart rate reserve and subjective exercise intensity (Borg scale) have been used for the exercise prescription (Fig. 5.2).

A prescription for the heart rate reserve uses Karvonen's formula: [maximum heart rate] − [resting heart rate] × k + resting heart rate. In mild- to moderate-HF cases (NYHA I to II), the target heart rate is set as $k = 0.4–0.5$, and in severe cases (NYHA III), the target heart rate is set as $k = 0.3–0.4$. In patients with HF who are taking β-blockers, the heart rate response during exercise is suppressed. The target rating of perceived exertion (RPE) is therefore set at Borg scale 11 (fairly light) to

13 (somewhat difficult). The exercise starts with a 5–10 min/session, 2 sessions/day, and then increases gradually to 20–30 min/session, 2 sessions/day. In mild cases of HF, exercise therapy is performed up to 5×/week, and in severe cases, it is performed 3×/week.

Exercise during the first month should be light in intensity and carefully monitored for worsening HF. The exercise program should start with supervised training; during the stable phase, this can be combined with non-supervised (home-based) exercise training. Changes in subjective symptoms, physical findings, body weight, and brain natriuretic peptide (BNP) levels should be observed.

Patients with HF are advised to perform daily activities with activities below the AT. For example, when the peak oxygen uptake at the AT is 10.5 mL/kg/min and the heart rate is 90/min by a cardiopulmonary exercise test, activity at a heart rate of approx. 90/min is acceptable. When the oxygen uptake at the patient's AT is divided by 3.5, the metabolic equivalents (METs) are calculated as 3. By using the daily life activity and METs correspondence table, it is possible to determine precisely how much activity can be performed without problems.

5.4 Sarcopenia in HF

Loss of muscle mass with aging was first proposed by Rosenberg in 1988 as sarcopenia. In 2010, the European Sarcopenia Working Group (EWGSOP) published a consensus on the diagnostic criteria for sarcopenia, stating that "Sarcopenia is associated with a risk of adverse outcomes such as physical disability, decreased QOL, and death, and is a progressive and generalized syndrome characterized by reduced skeletal muscle mass and strength." At age 50 and over, the body's skeletal muscle mass decreases by ~1%–2% per year, and 30% is lost by age 80. Sarcopenia is classified as primary or secondary. Primary sarcopenia shows no obvious causes other than aging; the causes of secondary sarcopenia include disuse, inflammation, malnutrition, organ failure, malignant tumor, inflammatory disease, endocrine disease, and other factors other than aging.

Sarcopenia is diagnosed in subjects with a decrease in muscle mass and muscle weakness or reduced physical function (Fig. 5.3) [6]. In the diagnostic criteria issued by the Asian Sarcopenia Working Group (AWGS), the dual energy X-ray absorption (DXA) method and bioelectric impedance (BIA) method are used to evaluate a subject's skeletal muscle mass. The limb lean mass or the limb skeletal muscle mass is measured and corrected by the square of the subject's height.

The overall prevalence of sarcopenia is reported to be 5%–13% between the ages of 65 and 70 and 11%–50% above the age of 80. In a study of 200 HF patients (mean age 69 ± 10 years, NYHA II–III), the frequency of sarcopenia complicated with HF was 19.5% [7]. A study using a sarcopenia score calculated based on the patient's age, grip strength, and lower-leg circumference reported that there were significantly more HF-related events in the HF patients with sarcopenia than in those without sarcopenia [8].

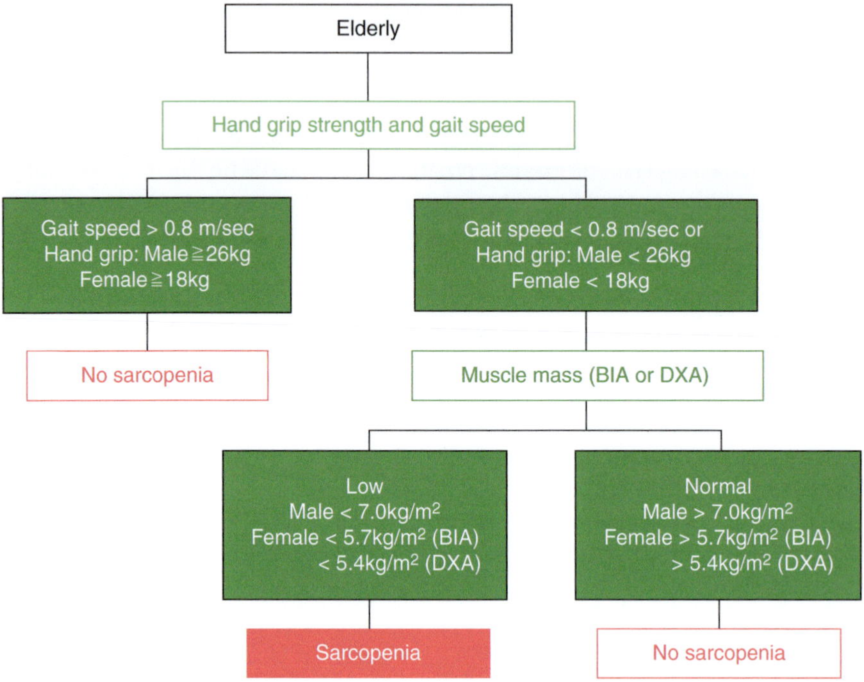

Fig. 5.3 The diagnostic criteria issued by the Asian Sarcopenia Working Group (AWGS). BIA: bioelectric impedance method, DXA: dual energy X-ray absorption method. Adapted from Ref. [6]

5.5 Resistance Exercise

Exercise is the most effective intervention for the prevention and improvement of sarcopenia because it has the effects of promoting anabolism of skeletal muscle and suppressing catabolism. In particular, resistance exercises using weight machines, free weights, rubber belts, or the body's own weight have been shown to increase muscle strength and muscle mass in many studies. It is known that a high-intensity load is necessary for muscle hypertrophy and muscle strength enhancement, but in HF patients, adverse events due to a high-intensity load occur frequently and close attention is required.

In HF patients with sarcopenia, combining low- to medium-intensity resistance exercise with systemic aerobic exercise is effective for improving exercise tolerance and QOL. In supervised exercise therapy, the resistance exercise should be performed 2–3×/week within the range of 20%–30% of the maximum load (1 repetition maximum: 1RM) or Borg scale 11 (fairly light) to 13 (somewhat hard). It is recommended that the range be gradually increased to 40%–60% 1RM. A study of healthy elderly people indicated that muscle mass and strength can be expected to increase by slow motions, even at low strength (30% 1RM), and that this can be applied to patients with HF [9]. Elderly people are known to lose muscle mass and strength even when they rest on a bed for a short period of time [10], and it is desirable that the elderly who are bedridden actively perform resistance exercises from the acute phase in order to prevent deconditioning.

The authors of a meta-analysis reported that neuromuscular electrical stimulation improved HF patients' peak oxygen uptake, 6 min walking distance, QOL, muscle strength, endothelial function, and depressive symptom. This may be an effective treatment for patients with complicated HF who cannot perform aerobic exercise [11].

5.6 Aerobic and Resistance Exercises in HF

As described above, both skeletal muscle atrophy/muscle weakness and reduced skeletal muscle endurance are present in patients with HF, and their underlying mechanisms are thought to differ. The effects of aerobic exercise and resistance exercise are also different. It is thus necessary to use aerobic exercise and resistance exercise in accord with the characteristics of each patient and the time of illness. At the stable phase and in cases without sarcopenia, exercise therapy is performed mainly with aerobic exercise. For patients during an early ambulation program [12] and for those who cannot perform endurance exercise (with frailty, orthopedic disease, neurological disease, etc.) resistance exercise should be introduced at an early stage, and the aim should be to maintain muscular strength as a minimum. Figure 5.4 provides a flowchart for exercise therapy.

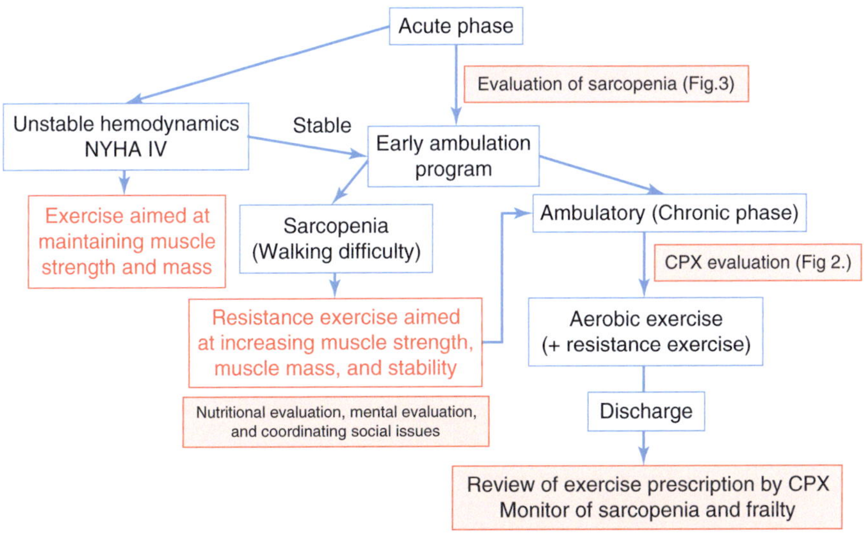

Fig. 5.4 Flow chart for exercise therapy. CPX: cardiopulmonary exercise test

5.7 Comprehensive Cardiac Rehabilitation

Many preventable factors (rather than medical factors) are known to be causes of rehospitalization due to worsening HF, including "incomplete salt and water restriction," "overwork," "mental stress," and "lack of medication adherence." When a patient with HF has been readmitted again, if the cause is not clarified and the countermeasures for the cause are not taken, rehospitalization is repeated. Disease management conducted by multi-professional teams has recently attracted attention, and its effects have been verified by many clinical trials. In J-HOMECARE, a randomized controlled trial that examined the effects of a disease management program on the psychological status, QOL score, mortality, and readmission in patients with chronic HF, the disease management program reduced depression and anxiety, improved the QOL, and decreased the rate of readmission due to exacerbation of HF [13].

Cardiac rehabilitation is a comprehensive program that provides not only exercise therapy but also life guidance, nutritional guidance, counseling, and patient education. In another study, post-discharge patients with HF were randomly assigned to a cardiac rehabilitation intervention group and a normal treatment group. In the intervention group, supervised exercise 1×/week, education guidance and HF checks by an HF specialist nurse, home-based exercise therapy guidance, and telephone consultation were performed for 3 months. The comprehensive cardiac rehabilitation improved the patients' QOL, increased their 6 min walking distance, and decreased the prevalence of severe HF (NYHA III and IV) after 1 year and the ratio of readmission for all causes. Comprehensive cardiac rehabilitation is considered a disease management program itself for chronic HF, and it is important for such programs to form multidisciplinary teams that include physicians, nurses, physical therapists, dietitians, pharmacists, and clinical psychologists.

References

1. Braunwald E, Bristow MR. Congestive heart failure: fifty years of progress. Circulation. 2000;102:IV14–23.
2. Tsutsui H, et al. JCS 2017/JHFS 2017 guideline on diagnosis and treatment of acute and chronic heart failure – digest version. Circ J. 2019;83:2084–184.
3. Belardinelli R, et al. Randomized, controlled trial of long-term moderate exercise training in chronic heart failure: effects on functional capacity, quality of life, and clinical outcome. Circulation. 1999;99:1173–82.
4. Piepoli MF, et al. Exercise training meta-analysis of trials in patients with chronic heart failure (ExTraMATCH). BMJ. 2004;328:189.
5. O'Connor CM, et al. Efficacy and safety of exercise training in patients with chronic heart failure: HF-ACTION randomized controlled trial. JAMA. 2009;301:1439–50.
6. Chen LK, et al. Sarcopenia in Asia: consensus report of the Asian Working Group for Sarcopenia. J Am Med Dir Assoc. 2014;15:95–101.
7. Fulster S, et al. Muscle wasting in patients with chronic heart failure: results from the studies investigating co-morbidities aggravating heart failure (SICA-HF). Eur Heart J. 2013;34:512–9.

8. Kamiya K, et al. Prognostic usefulness of arm and calf circumference in patients ≥65 years of age with cardiovascular disease. Am J Cardiol. 2016;119(2):186–91. https://doi.org/10.1010/j.amjcard.016.09.040.
9. Watanabe Y, et al. Effect of very low-intensity resistance training with slow movement on muscle size and strength in healthy older adults. Clin Physiol Funct Imaging. 2014;34:463–70.
10. Kortebein P, et al. Effect of 10 days of bed rest on skeletal muscle in healthy older adults. JAMA. 2007;297:1772–4.
11. Gomes Neto M, et al. Effects of neuromuscular electrical stimulation on physiologic and functional measurements in patients with heart failure: a systematic review with meta-analysis. J Cardiopulm Rehabil Prev. 2016;36:157–66.
12. Izawa H, et al. Standard cardiac rehabilitation program for heart failure. Circ J. 2019;83:2394–8.
13. Tsuchihashi-Makaya M, et al. Home-based disease management program to improve psychological status in patients with heart failure in Japan. Circ J. 2013;77:926–33.

Chapter 6
IABP/ECMO

Takeo Fujino

Abstract Intra-aortic balloon pump (IABP) has been the most common mechanical circulatory support device for a cardiogenic shock for a long time, with its easy and safety profile. Recently, the strategies are changing based on large clinical trials. The use of veno-arterial extracorporeal membrane oxygenation (VA-ECMO) for refractory cardiogenic shock is rapidly increasing, with the improvement of device technology and practical management. VA-ECMO can achieve complete cardiopulmonary support with remarkable improvement of systemic perfusion if we can manage its hemodynamic changes and associated complications. This chapter describes the overview, current evidence, and clinical practice of IABP and ECMO therapies.

Keywords Intra-aortic balloon pump · Veno-arterial extracorporeal membrane oxygenation · Cardiogenic shock · Mechanical support · Hemodynamics · Indication · Complication

6.1 IABP

6.1.1 Overview

Treatment with an intra-aortic balloon pump (IABP) was first reported in 1968, and after that it has become the most common form of mechanical circulatory support for the failing heart [1]. With a balloon placed in the descending aorta, inflation of the balloon in diastole and active deflation in systole induce "volume displacement" of blood within the aorta at both proximal and distal locations. This action leads to a potential increase in coronary blood flow and an improvement in systemic perfusion, as well as a decrease in left ventricle (LV) afterload, although the hemodynamic effect is relatively small. Hemodynamic effects expected with IABP are listed below (Table 6.1):

T. Fujino (✉)
Department of Medicine, Section of Cardiology, University of Chicago Medicine, Chicago, IL, USA
e-mail: tafujino@cardiol.med.kyushu-u.ac.jp

K. Kinugawa, T. Imamura (eds.), *Update of Non-Pharmacological Therapy for Heart Failure*, https://doi.org/10.1007/978-981-15-4843-7_6

Table 6.1 Hemodynamic effect of IABP and VA-ECMO

Device	IABP	VA-ECMO
Mean aortic pressure	Increase	Increase
LV preload	Decrease	Increase
LV afterload	Decrease	Increase
Stroke volume	Increase	Decrease
Coronary perfusion	Increase	(Increase?)
Peripheral tissue perfusion	Increase	Increase
Myocardial oxygen demand	Decrease	Increase

- An increase in stroke volume and cardiac output (by 0.5–1.0 L/min)
- An increase in diastolic blood pressure with a potential increase in coronary blood flow
- A decrease in LV preload
- A decrease in LV afterload
- A decrease in myocardial oxygen demand

6.1.2 *IABP for Cardiogenic Shock (CS): Current Evidence*

6.1.2.1 Definition of CS

CS is a state in which ineffective cardiac output caused by a primary cardiac disorder results in both clinical and biochemical manifestations of inadequate tissue perfusion. The clinical presentation is typically characterized by persistent hypotension unresponsive to volume replacement and is accompanied by clinical features of end-organ hypoperfusion requiring intervention with pharmacological and/or mechanical support. There are a number of causes of CS, including acute myocardial infarction, chronic heart failure with decompensation, acute myocarditis, peripartum cardiomyopathy, and post-cardiotomy shock. Commonly accepted hemodynamic parameters defining CS include systolic blood pressure < 90 mmHg, cardiac index < 2.2 L/min/m^2, and pulmonary capillary wedge pressure > 15 mmHg [2]. Recovery is rare with pharmacological therapy alone and mechanical circulatory support is often required.

6.1.2.2 IABP for CS

In 2013, the largest randomized controlled trial in patients with CS after acute myocardial infarction (AMI) demonstrated neither benefit nor harm of the IABP therapy [3]. The findings have led to a paradigm shift away from routine IABP use in these cohorts. A guideline from European Society of Cardiology suggests that routine use of IABP for CS as a Class III recommendation [4].

CS is recently recognized as a condition with a spectrum with varying etiologies, phenotypes, and degrees of severity [5]. For example, in chronic heart failure (HF) patients with acute decompensation and CS may represent a different physiologic phenotype compared with AMI population. Some reports have shown the clinical utility of IABP in such patients [6, 7]. Others also reported that the acute hemodynamic improvement with IABP compared with inotropes in chronic HF patients [8]. Furthermore, considering its physiological effect, IABP can be more effective in CS patients with acute mitral regurgitation or a ventricular septal defect [9]. Even though the routine use of IABP for AMI with CS patients is not recommended, further studies are still expected to figure out the utility of IABP in carefully selected specific cohorts.

6.1.3 Clinical Practice and Future Perspective

Before insertion, an appropriate balloon size should be selected on the basis of the patient's height. The balloon catheter is inserted and advanced, usually under fluoroscopic guidance, to the descending thoracic aorta, where its proximal tip is positioned 2–3 cm distal to the origin of the left subclavian artery (at the level of the carina). The distal balloon end should be positioned above the renal arteries. Incorrect balloon position results in reduced diastolic augmentation or vascular complications due to intimal injury, plaque distortion, or direct occlusion of the arterial lumen.

Generally, IABP is inserted from a femoral artery; however, patients with femoral IABP have restricted mobilization, limiting the duration of support into days to weeks. Recently, the safety and efficacy of subclavian IABP was reported, which enabled patients' mobilization and then longer term IABP support [10]. Furthermore, an implantable device with intra-aortic counterpulsation through the subclavian artery was also proposed recently [11, 12]. Longer term ambulatory IABP can be a novel strategy for advanced HF and CS patients in the near future.

IABP is contraindicated in patients with significant aortic regurgitation because it worsens regurgitation. IABP device insertion should not be attempted in a patient with suspected or known aortic dissection. Aortic rupture is a potential consequence of IABP device insertion in patients with aortic dissection or aortic aneurysms. IABP device placement should be avoided in patients with severe peripheral vascular disease. IABP may be associated with vascular complications, including bleeding, systemic embolization, limb ischemia, and amputation. In addition, as with any indwelling catheter, IABP may cause systemic infection. The presence of a fever in a patient with IABP, in the absence of another clear source, requires balloon removal. In a large multinational registry, 7.0% of IABP recipients experienced IABP-related complications. Of them, 2.6% had major vascular complications, including severe access site bleeding in 0.8%, major limb ischemia in 0.9%, limb amputation in 0.1%, and IABP-related mortality in 0.05% [13].

6.2 Veno-arterial Extracorporeal Membrane Oxygenation (VA-ECMO)

6.2.1 Overview

Extracorporeal membrane oxygenation (ECMO) offers pulmonary or cardiopulmonary support depending on its configuration of cannulation sites (Fig. 6.1). ECMO was used primarily in neonatology, predominantly as a veno-venous (VV)-ECMO. VV-ECMO was first used in adults with severe but potentially reversible lung disease. In contrast, veno-arterial (VA)-ECMO provides both gas exchange and circulatory support through a continuous-flow pump. It can be used in the setting of left ventricular or biventricular failure, complicated with respiratory failure. Since its introduction in 1972, national trends demonstrate a substantial increase in peripheral VA-ECMO use for refractory CS. Especially it is rapidly increasing in recent years with the improvement in device technology and practical management [14].

In principle, VA-ECMO drains venous blood through a cannula and returns it to the artery via another cannula into the body, driven by a centrifugal pump. During ECMO passage the blood becomes oxygenated, decarboxylated, and warmed in an extracorporeal gas exchange unit. The hemodynamic effects of VA-ECMO are shown in Table 6.1. VA-ECMO drains and returns up to 6.0 L/

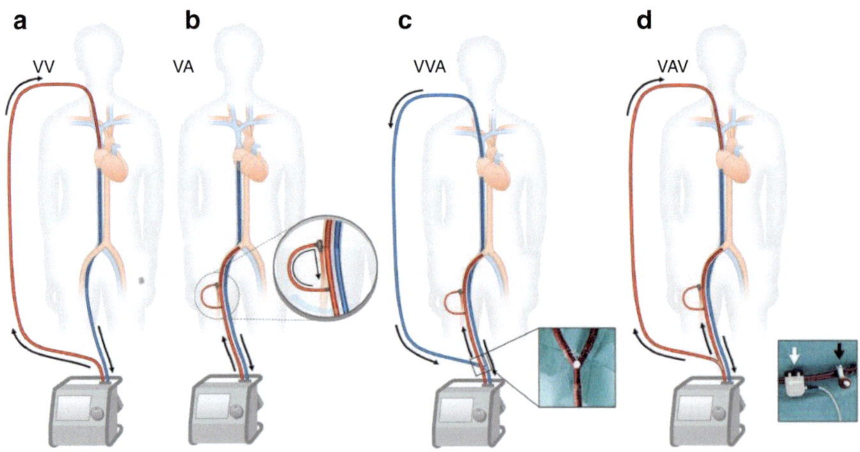

Fig. 6.1 Various configurations of ECMO. (**a**) Veno-venous (VV)-ECMO with femoral and jugular vein cannulation. (**b**) Veno-arterial (VA)-ECMO with femoral artery/vein cannulation and antegrade perfusion. (**c**) Veno-veno-arterial (VVA)-ECMO with femoral artery/vein and jugular vein cannulation and antegrade perfusion. (**d**) Veno-arterio-venous (VAV)-ECMO with femoral artery/vein and jugular vein cannulation and antegrad perfusion. Modified from Napp et al. [21]

min of flow, which effectively reduces right ventricular (RV) preload and improves end-organ perfusion, but it enhances LV afterload, which causes an increase of LV preload and exacerbates pulmonary edema. It also decreases stroke volume, and increase myocardial oxygen demand. The effect of VA-ECMO on coronary perfusion varies based on multiple factors. Increased aortic pressure may improve coronary perfusion; in contrast, an increase of LV end-diastolic pressure may reduce the trans-coronary perfusion gradient and can impair coronary perfusion.

These hemodynamic responses to VA-ECMO can be modulated by other factors. A reduction in LV afterload during ECMO markedly blunts the rise in LV preload. Therefore, unloading of LV is important to avoid pulmonary edema, and also to improve coronary perfusion and accelerate cardiac recovery. There are several strategies for unloading LV during VA-ECMO. Of them, IABP or Impella (ECMO + Impella, ECPELLA) are recently used concurrently with VA-ECMO [15, 16]. Improvements in LV function can also modulate the rise in LV preload. LV function can be improved during ECMO due to elevated aortic pressure (and coronary perfusion), normalization of blood oxygen content, and improvement of acid–base and other metabolic abnormalities [17].

6.2.2 *VA-ECMO for CS: Current Evidence*

As noted above, the clinical efficacy of IABP in patients with CS after AMI was not proved in a large clinical trial [3]. Other short-term mechanical support devices such as Impella and Tandem Heart did not show superiority compared to IABP [18]. Evidence favoring adult VA-ECMO came from prospective observational propensity-matched studies of extracorporeal cardiopulmonary resuscitation, both demonstrating a neurologically intact survival benefit over conventional cardiopulmonary resuscitation. However, there are no randomized data supporting the effectiveness of VA-ECMO in patients with refractory CS thus far [19].

Nevertheless, a number of previous studies have suggested the effectiveness of VA-ECMO in various types of CS. Survival to discharge ranges from 19.2% to 87.5% in CS due to acute myocardial infarction, from 47% to 83.3% for myocarditis, and 57% to 100% for pulmonary embolism. Of note, two groups of patients, those with fulminant myocarditis and those with pulmonary embolism had excellent reported survival [14].

The superiority of ECMO than other devices is the ability to simultaneously biventricular support and to provide oxygenation; the management can be easier than biventricular assist devices. Furthermore, the time to cannulation is generally shorter than other percutaneous devices such as Impella 5.0 or Tandem Heart.

6.2.3 Indications and Contraindications

Generally, VA-ECMO is indicated in these conditions: (1) cardiac arrest; (2) refractory CS; (3) refractory ventricular tachycardia; (4) RV failure during LVAD support; and (5) failure to wean off cardiopulmonary bypass. Because the duration of ECMO support is limited for days to weeks dominantly due to its complications, the key to ECMO success is the use of ECMO as a "bridge therapy" to recovery or definitive treatment. ECMO does not cure the underlying condition; it provides time to treat underlying conditions or to find a long-term solution, such as durable left ventricular assist devices (LVAD). In other words, the purpose of VA-ECMO insertion is: (1) bridge to recovery; provide circulatory support while the heart recovers, spontaneously or with treatment; (2) bridge to decision; determine reversibility of end-organ damage after a catastrophic or critical myocardial event; (3) bridge to bridge; achieve a period of temporary stability until durable device therapy. Lack of a solution or a potential to recovery should discourage ECMO initiation.

Absolute contraindications for ECMO include severe irreversible noncardiac organ failure limiting survival (e.g., devastating stroke/anoxic brain injury, end-stage liver/kidney dysfunction, and advanced cancer), irreversible cardiac failure if durable LVAD is not considered, and aortic dissection. Relative contraindication includes older age, severe coagulopathy or contraindication to anticoagulation, limited vascular access, and significant aortic regurgitation.

Various predictors of mortality on VA-ECMO were proposed previously. Data from the International Extracorporeal Life Support Organization (ELSO) registry showed that chronic renal failure, longer duration of ventilation prior to ECMO initiation, pre-ECMO organ failures, pre-ECMO cardiac arrest, congenital heart disease, lower arterial pulse pressure, and lower serum bicarbonate were risk factors associated with mortality during ECMO support. In contrast, younger age, lower weight, acute myocarditis, heart transplant, refractory ventricular tachyarrhythmia, higher diastolic blood pressure, and lower peak inspiratory pressure were protective factors. Based on the results, SAVE-score was created and can be a tool to predict survival for patients receiving VA-ECMO for refractory CS [20].

6.2.4 Clinical Practice

6.2.4.1 Cannulation

Peripheral VA-ECMO is established percutaneously in the catheterization laboratory or at the bedside. In less urgent situations, surgical cut-down in the operating room may be considered to avoid the risk of bleeding, infection, and vascular complications. For percutaneous insertion, ultrasonographic evaluation of the vessels should be performed to determine the size of cannulas and assist initial needle insertion.

The amount of flow generated is largely dependent on the size of the cannulas. Although the ideal size of cannulas for arterial and venous cannulation has not been clearly defined so far, larger cannulas are generally recommended for adequate hemodynamic support. For adult patients, our institutional protocol recommends 23–27 Fr for venous and 17–21 Fr for arterial cannulation.

There are several variations of VA-ECMO configuration based on the type of cannulation (Fig. 6.1). In nonsurgical applications in adults, peripheral cannulation of the femoral artery and vein is the standard technique. In surgical application, we can also choose direct cannulation to right atrium and aorta via sternotomy (central VA-ECMO), or cannulation to the jugular vein and axillary artery, which enables patients' mobilization with VA-ECMO. Although it requires sternotomy, central VA-ECMO can provide sufficient amount of ECMO flow with larger arterial and venous cannulas than peripheral VA-ECMO. Generally it is technically easier to establish central VA-ECMO than paracorporeal biventricular assist device, which requires cannulation into the ventricles. In addition, the management of central VA-ECMO is easier than biventricular assist device because it does not need to adjust the balance of left and right pumps. We can also unload the LV by addition of direct venting cannulation.

If VA-ECMO does not generate adequate flow, the reason for inadequate flow often results from small venous cannula. We can resolve this situation by adding another venous draining cannula (VVA-ECMO), or changing to central VA-ECMO with larger cannulas.

As the LV myocardium recovers, it starts ejecting the blood that LV receives from the pulmonary circulation. Forward flow of deoxygenated blood from failing native lungs mixes unpredictably with retrograde flow from the oxygenator, which can result in inadequate delivery of oxygenated blood into the aortic arch. This phenomenon, known as Harlequin syndrome, north-south syndrome, or differential hypoxia, may result in hypoxia of the coronary arteries, upper extremities, and brain. In such cases, we can add another venous cannula and blood returns to both artery and vein, which can improve oxygenation of blood through the lung (VAV-ECMO) [21].

6.2.4.2 Daily Management

Daily close monitoring is a key to obtain adequate hemodynamic support, avoid serious complications, and subsequently achieve a therapeutic goal. A combination of team members such as ECMO specialists, nurses, physicians, and surgeons is essential for close monitoring of ECMO patients. To obtain adequate hemodynamics during VA-ECMO support, we typically set the target ECMO flow as 2.4 L/min/m^2, but more flow may be required in case of higher oxygen demand such as infection. A Swan-Ganz catheter should be placed and used as a tool to monitor pulmonary arterial pressure as a surrogate of LV distention. Adequate peripheral perfusion should be closely monitored by physical examination, urine volume, and intermittent measurement of mixed venous saturation, lactate, and end-organ function.

Systemic anticoagulation therapy is essential to prevent thrombus formation. The choice of agent used for anticoagulation, as well as monitoring of the level of anticoagulation, varies from site to site. Heparin is the most common anticoagulant, monitored by the activated partial thromboplastin time with a target goal 50 to 75 sec or 1.5-folds to 2.5-folds of baseline. Some centers prefer to follow the activated clotting time given its bedside availability and rapid turnaround time. Direct thrombin inhibitors such as argatroban represent alternatives to heparin in individuals with heparin-induced thrombocytopenia [14].

Recently, the implication of aggressive early rehabilitation during ECMO support is discussed. Early mobilization may prevent muscle weakness (ICU-acquired weakness) and reduce the risk of pulmonary complications such as pneumonia. We start mobilization protocol of VA-ECMO patients as soon as possible, and coordination of multidisciplinary team members is a key to success. Previous reports have suggested the safety of mobilization even for the patients with femoral VA-ECMO; however, converting cannulation sites from femoral artery/vein to upper body (jugular vein, axillary artery, or central ECMO) makes mobilization easier [22]. Further studies are expected to investigate the clinical implication of early rehabilitation in VA-ECMO patients.

6.2.4.3 Weaning

If patient hemodynamics improves on VA-ECMO, weaning is the next step. The candidate for weaning should have recovered a pulsatile arterial waveform for at least 24 h, should have baseline mean arterial pressure greater than 60 mmHg in the absence or with low doses of catecholamine, and should have recovered from major metabolic disturbances. Pulmonary function should also be confirmed to be improved. There is no standardized protocol for weaning, but some reports recommend a stepwise reduction of pump flow 0.5 L every 6–24 h [23]. The patient should be able to maintain a mixed venous saturation > 65% and an arterial saturation of >90% with a weaning trial of ECMO flow 1.0–1.5 L/min. If LV recovery were not sufficient for ECMO removal, bridging to other devices such as Impella is another option. If the pulmonary function were severely impaired, we should consider bridging to VV-ECMO [24].

6.2.5 Complications

A meta-analysis showed that limb ischemia developed in 16.9% of patients supported by peripheral VA-ECMO. Fasciotomy, due to compartment syndrome, was needed in 10.3% of patients, with 4.7% requiring amputation [25]. The use of prophylactic antegrade perfusion catheters has reduced the incidence of this complication and currently, it is strongly recommended [26]. We generally use 8 Fr sheath for antegrade perfusion and distal flow is monitored and maintained to >0.15 L/min. Typical symptoms of limb ischemia include pallor, loss of pulses, and gangrene. Compartment syndrome is rarely seen in profoundly ischemic limbs before reperfusion; after reperfusion, however, the limb may become swollen. If the measurement of the compartment pressures reveals a value above 20 mmHg, fasciotomy is usually required [14]. A high index of suspicion is necessary as are frequent Doppler checks and hourly monitoring. The presence of an elevated creatinine phosphokinase or lactate level is usually a late and very concerning finding.

Ischemic and hemorrhagic strokes occur in approximately 5.9% of VA-ECMO patients [25]. The previous study showed that cannulation via an axillary artery or ascending aorta (central VA-ECMO) did not increase the risk of stroke compared with femoral artery cannulation [27]. The cognitive function should be monitored continuously in ECMO patients. The cause of stroke is multifactorial, with thromboembolic events, systemic anticoagulation, and hemodynamic instability thought to contribute. Because of the low-flow state, thrombi can form spontaneously in the LA and LV. They can also form in the ECMO circuit.

Patients on VA-ECMO are anticoagulated and so prone to bleeding and 40% of patients experience any significant bleedings. Bleeding is treated by reducing or stopping anticoagulation. The previous study suggested that it is safe to withdraw anticoagulation in a select group of patients with coagulation abnormalities or bleeding [28]. Conversion to central VA-ECMO is highly recommended in case of uncontrollable complications associated with peripheral cannulation, such as limb ischemia and bleeding from the cannulation site.

Infectious complications such as ventilator-associated pneumonia and catheter or cannula-related bacteremia are also common in patients with VA-ECMO. Longer duration of ECMO is associated with a higher risk of infection. Infectious complications are significantly associated with higher mortality.

References

1. Kantrowitz A, Tjonneland S, Freed PS, et al. Initial clinical experience with intraaortic balloon pumping in cardiogenic shock. JAMA. 1968;203(2):113–8.
2. Hochman JS, Sleeper LA, Webb JG, et al. Early revascularization in acute myocardial infarction complicated by cardiogenic shock. SHOCK Investigators. Should we emergently revascularize occluded coronaries for cardiogenic shock. N Engl J Med. 1999;341(9):625–34.
3. Thiele H, Zeymer U, Neumann FJ, et al. Intra-aortic balloon counterpulsation in acute myocardial infarction complicated by cardiogenic shock (IABP-SHOCK II): final 12 month results of a randomised, open-label trial. Lancet. 2013;382(9905):1638–45.
4. Ponikowski P, Voors AA, Anker SD, et al. 2016 ESC guidelines for the diagnosis and treatment of acute and chronic heart failure: the task force for the diagnosis and treatment of acute and chronic heart failure of the European Society of Cardiology (ESC) developed with the special contribution of the Heart Failure Association (HFA) of the ESC. Eur Heart J. 2016;37(27):2129–200.

5. Baran DA, Grines CL, Bailey S, et al. SCAI clinical expert consensus statement on the classification of cardiogenic shock: this document was endorsed by the American College of Cardiology (ACC), the American Heart Association (AHA), the Society of Critical Care Medicine (SCCM), and the Society of Thoracic Surgeons (STS) in April 2019. Catheter Cardiovasc Interv. 2019;94(1):29–37.
6. Fried JA, Nair A, Takeda K, et al. Clinical and hemodynamic effects of intra-aortic balloon pump therapy in chronic heart failure patients with cardiogenic shock. J Heart Lung Transplant. 2018;37(11):1313–21.
7. Sintek MA, Gdowski M, Lindman BR, et al. Intra-aortic balloon counterpulsation in patients with chronic heart failure and cardiogenic shock: clinical response and predictors of stabilization. J Card Fail. 2015;21(11):868–76.
8. den Uil CA, Van Mieghem NM, Bastos MB, et al. Primary intra-aortic balloon support versus inotropes for decompensated heart failure and low output: a randomised trial. EuroIntervention. 2019;15(7):586–93.
9. van Diepen S, Katz JN, Albert NM, et al. Contemporary management of cardiogenic shock: a scientific statement from the American Heart Association. Circulation. 2017;136(16):e232–68.
10. Tanaka A, Tuladhar SM, Onsager D, et al. The subclavian intraaortic balloon pump: a compelling bridge device for advanced heart failure. Ann Thorac Surg. 2015;100(6):2151–7.. discussion 2157–2158
11. Imamura T, Juricek C, Song T, et al. Improvement in biventricular cardiac function after ambulatory counterpulsation. J Card Fail. 2019;25(1):20–6.
12. Jeevanandam V, Song T, Onsager D, et al. The first-in-human experience with a minimally invasive, ambulatory, counterpulsation heart assist system for advanced congestive heart failure. J Heart Lung Transplant. 2018;37(1):1–6.
13. Ferguson JJ 3rd, Cohen M, Freedman RJ Jr, et al. The current practice of intra-aortic balloon counterpulsation: results from the benchmark registry. J Am Coll Cardiol. 2001;38(5):1456–62.
14. Guglin M, Zucker MJ, Bazan VM, et al. Venoarterial ECMO for adults: JACC Scientific Expert Panel. J Am Coll Cardiol. 2019;73(6):698–716.
15. Rao P, Khalpey Z, Smith R, et al. Venoarterial extracorporeal membrane oxygenation for cardiogenic shock and cardiac arrest. Circ Heart Fail. 2018;11(9):e004905.
16. Russo JJ, Aleksova N, Pitcher I, et al. Left ventricular unloading during extracorporeal membrane oxygenation in patients with cardiogenic shock. J Am Coll Cardiol. 2019;73(6):654–62.
17. Burkhoff D, Sayer G, Doshi D, et al. Hemodynamics of mechanical circulatory support. J Am Coll Cardiol. 2015;66(23):2663–74.
18. Thiele H, Jobs A, Ouweneel DM, et al. Percutaneous short-term active mechanical support devices in cardiogenic shock: a systematic review and collaborative meta-analysis of randomized trials. Eur Heart J. 2017;38(47):3523–31.
19. Chen YS, Lin JW, Yu HY, et al. Cardiopulmonary resuscitation with assisted extracorporeal life-support versus conventional cardiopulmonary resuscitation in adults with in-hospital cardiac arrest: an observational study and propensity analysis. Lancet. 2008;372(9638):554–61.
20. Schmidt M, Burrell A, Roberts L, et al. Predicting survival after ECMO for refractory cardiogenic shock: the survival after veno-arterial-ECMO (SAVE)-score. Eur Heart J. 2015;36(33):2246–56.
21. Napp LC, Kuhn C, Hoeper MM, et al. Cannulation strategies for percutaneous extracorporeal membrane oxygenation in adults. Clin Res Cardiol. 2016;105(4):283–96.
22. Wells CL, Forrester J, Vogel J, et al. Safety and feasibility of early physical therapy for patients on extracorporeal membrane oxygenator: University of Maryland Medical Center experience. Crit Care Med. 2018;46(1):53–9.
23. Pappalardo F, Pieri M, Arnaez Corada B, et al. Timing and strategy for weaning from venoarterial ECMO are complex issues. J Cardiothorac Vasc Anesth. 2015;29(4):906–11.
24. Aissaoui N, El-Banayosy A, Combes A. How to wean a patient from veno-arterial extracorporeal membrane oxygenation. Intensive Care Med. 2015;41(5):902–5.

25. Cheng R, Hachamovitch R, Kittleson M, et al. Complications of extracorporeal membrane oxygenation for treatment of cardiogenic shock and cardiac arrest: a meta-analysis of 1,866 adult patients. Ann Thorac Surg. 2014;97(2):610–6.
26. Juo YY, Skancke M, Sanaiha Y, et al. Efficacy of distal perfusion Cannulae in preventing limb ischemia during extracorporeal membrane oxygenation: a systematic review and meta-analysis. Artif Organs. 2017;41(11):E263–73.
27. Ranney DN, Benrashid E, Meza JM, et al. Central cannulation as a viable alternative to peripheral cannulation in extracorporeal membrane oxygenation. Semin Thorac Cardiovasc Surg. 2017;29(2):188–95.
28. Chung YS, Cho DY, Sohn DS, et al. Is stopping heparin safe in patients on extracorporeal membrane oxygenation treatment? ASAIO J. 2017;63(1):32–6.

Chapter 7
Impella

Makiko Nakamura and Koichiro Kinugawa

Abstract Impella (Abiomed, Danvers, MA, USA) is a recently innovated micro-axial flow pump which is inserted percutaneously and transfers blood from the left ventricle to the ascending aorta, improving systemic circulation and end-organ dysfunction and unloading left ventricle in patients with cardiogenic shock. Impella has not shown a significant survival benefit in patients with cardiogenic shock compared with conventional intra-aortic balloon pumping in the randomized control trials. However, given powerful and immediate circulatory support, Impella would be a promising tool as bridge to durable mechanical circulatory support devices or as bridge to recovery.

Keywords Cardiogenic shock · Temporary mechanical circulatory support · Mechanical unloading · Bridge to recovery · Bridge to decision

7.1 Impella Left Ventricular Support System

The Impella left ventricular assist device family (Abiomed, Danvers, MA, USA; Table 7.1) is inserted fluoroscopically into the left ventricle via aortic valve in retrograde fashion through the femoral artery or axillary artery. As of November 2019, Impella 2.5, CP, and 5.0 have been approved and commercially available in Japan.

The distal portion of the Impella is a pigtail configuration (Fig. 7.1a) that is meant to reside in the mid left ventricle (LV) approximately 3.5 cm below the aortic annulus and its length varies slightly depending on the type of Impella (Fig. 7.1b).

M. Nakamura (✉) · K. Kinugawa
The Second Department of Internal Medicine, University of Toyama, Toyama, Japan

K. Kinugawa, T. Imamura (eds.), *Update of Non-Pharmacological Therapy for Heart Failure*, https://doi.org/10.1007/978-981-15-4843-7_7

Blood is drawn from the inlet (located just superior to the catheter's pigtail in the LV cavity) and delivered through the Impella outlet, which is seated just above the aortic valve (Fig. 7.1a).

A pressure barrier is formed with pressurized heparinized glucose solution (purge solution) so that blood does not enter the motor pump catheter. This system is called "purge system."

Table 7.1 Types of Impella

	2.5	CP	5.0
Max flow (L/min)	2.5 L/min	3.7 L/min	5.0 L/min
Maximum rotation speed (rpm)	51,000	46,000	33,000
Pump size (Fr)	12 Fr	14 Fr	21 Fr
Placement	Perc (puncture)	Perc (puncture)	Perc (cut down)
Insertion site	Femoral	Femoral	Axillary
Effective length of left ventricle	7.5 cm	8.5 cm	7.0 cm
Duration of support	Hours to days	Days	Days to weeks

Fr French, *Perc* Percutaneous

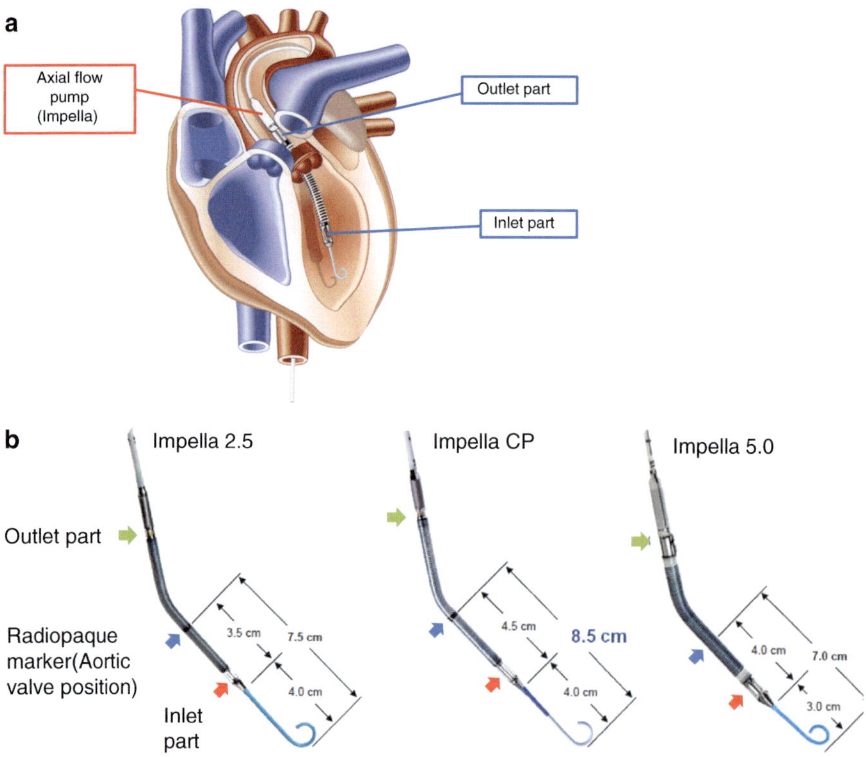

Fig. 7.1 (**a**) Overview of Impella. (**b**) Length that requires insertion of the Impella pump catheter into the left ventricle

7.2 Indication, Background, and Complication of Impella

The Impella devices have been used in various clinical situations, including cardiogenic shock with ST-elevation myocardial infarction (STEMI), acute on chronic decompensated heart failure dominantly due to dilated cardiomyopathy or ischemic cardiomyopathy, or fulminant myocarditis (Fig. 7.2).

It has been reported that the clinical outcome was superior in 30-day mortality in patients with cardiogenic shock due to STEMI when Impella was inserted before percutaneous coronary intervention (PCI) compared with those inserted after PCI [1]. Furthermore, it has been reported that LV unloading by Impella before PCI reduced reperfusion injury as well as the infarcted myocardial size and improved cardiac function [2].

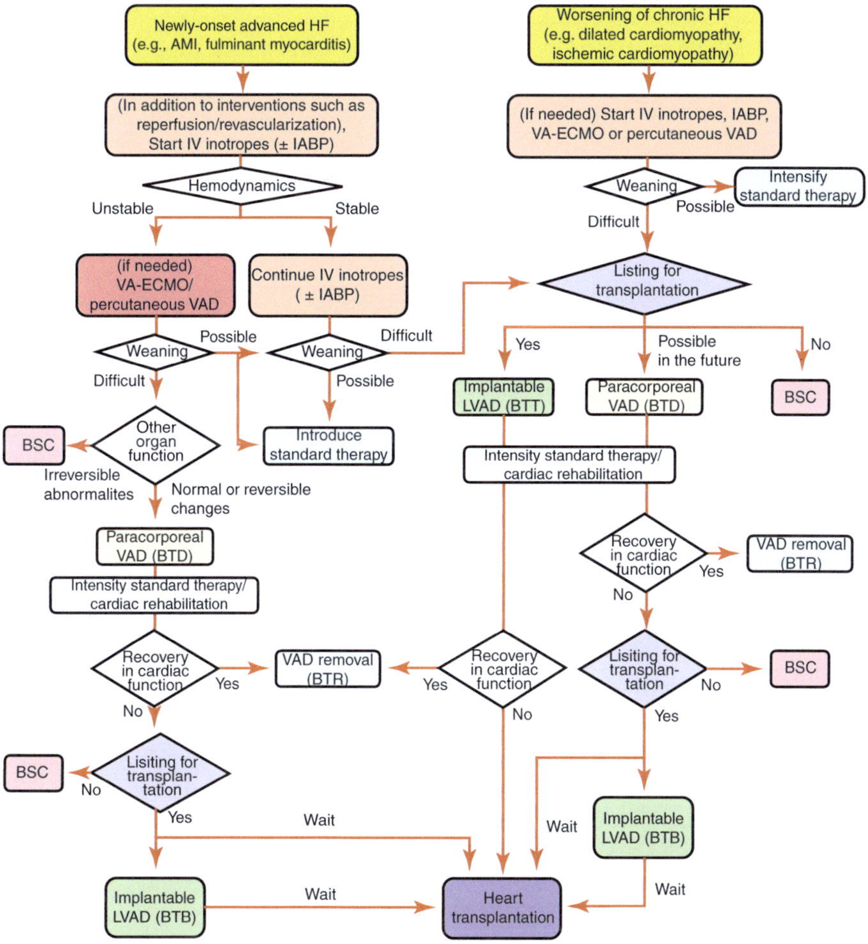

Fig. 7.2 The standing position of Impella (percutaneous VAD) in the treatment of advanced HF. *HF* heart failure

Several small-scale randomized clinical trials could not show a survival benefit of Impella over the intra-aortic balloon pumping despite superiority in improving hemodynamics [3, 4]. Of note, most trials of temporary mechanical circulatory support (TCS) were conducted in small cohorts. Furthermore, the timing of TCS initiation was not clearly stated or defined in these clinical trials. Impella 5.0 can provide superior LV unloading and higher systemic flows compared to the conventional devices, whereas it has not yet been evaluated in the prospective randomized trials. A recent meta-analysis examining the outcome of Impella 5.0 among a total of 163 patients with cardiogenic shock demonstrated 73.5% of survival to discharge and a high rate of myocardial recovery [5]. Impella 5.0 also provides a bridge to decision strategy for patients with advanced heart failure and acute hemodynamic instability [6].

The following complications are known; hemolysis and pigment-induced nephropathy, vascular access complications (e.g., limb ischemia and major bleeding), infection, mitral valve impingement with mitral regurgitation, and device failure due to thrombosis. The positive hemodynamic effect provided by the Impella might be neutralized by the higher incidence of peripheral vascular complications, severe or life-threatening bleedings, and infections, in the large-scale clinical trials [7]. Improvements in the device technology and peri-procedural management to reduce such comorbidities might clarify the actual clinical benefit of Impella therapy.

7.3 ECPELLA (ECMO Plus Impella)

In cases of ventricular tachycardia/ventricular fibrillation or any other critical hemodynamic deterioration complicated with STEMI, not only LV support with Impella but also right ventricle (RV) and oxygenation supports are required, and extracorporeal membrane oxygenation (ECMO) is concomitantly used together with Impella targeting synergetic effects of both devices (i.e., ECPELLA). In cases of fulminant myocarditis with additional severe impairment of the RV, ECMO has frequently been used. However, ECMO increases systemic afterload, LV filling pressures, and pulmonary capillary pressures due to the blood return to the central artery. The increased systemic afterload and cardiac filling pressure can be reduced by concomitantly used Impella [8]. It is reported that THE survival was better when supported by ECPELLA system than ECMO support alone in 30-day mortality in patients with refractory cardiogenic shock [9]. Recently, various favorable clinical outcomes of Impella or ECPELLA support have been reported particularly in patients with acute fulminant myocarditis [8, 10].

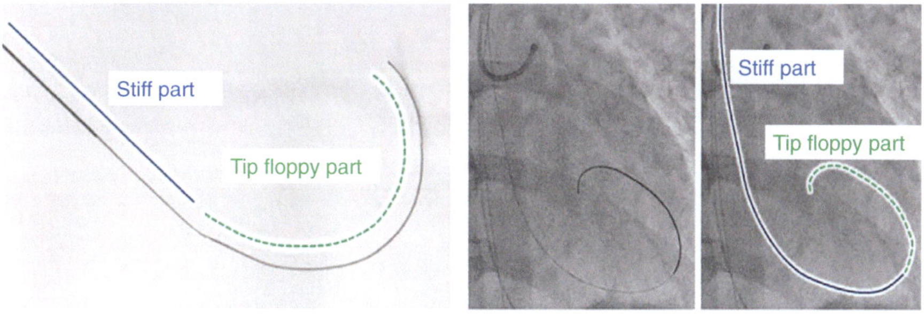

Add a large J curve to the tip of the floppy part (7cm)

Insert the indwelling guidewire so that it arches at the apex. The stiff part becomes a rail to ensure that the pump catheter can be guided toward the apex.

Fig. 7.3 The method of Impella (guidewire) insertion to the left ventricle

7.4 The Methodology of Impella Delivery into the Left Ventricle

The Impella indwelling guidewire is inserted into the LV so that it arches at the apex, after adding a large J curve to the tip of the floppy part. The stiff part of the guidewire becomes as a rail and can guide the Impella pump catheter toward the apex (Fig. 7.3).

7.5 Management Practice During Impella Support

After Impella insertion, mean arterial pressure would increase and pulse pressure would decrease. Optimal mean arterial pressure is above 70 mmHg and less than 90 mmHg. There are three points to be confirmed as following: (1) The positioning of Impella pump catheter; (2) Bleeding at the puncture site and others; and (3) Improvement of end-organ function and pulmonary congestion. Especially in patients with Impella inserted via femoral artery, we should confirm and adjust the position of the Impella pump catheter by echocardiography at least once a day.

At the time of Impella insertion, activated clotting time (ACT) >250 s should be required. To maintain Impella system, ACT should not be longer than 200 s to avoid critical bleeding. The heparin concentration of the purge solution is initiated at 10–20 units/mL at first and is gradually increased to maintain ACT 170–180 s and APTT 50–60 s after confirmation of the hemostasis at the puncture site.

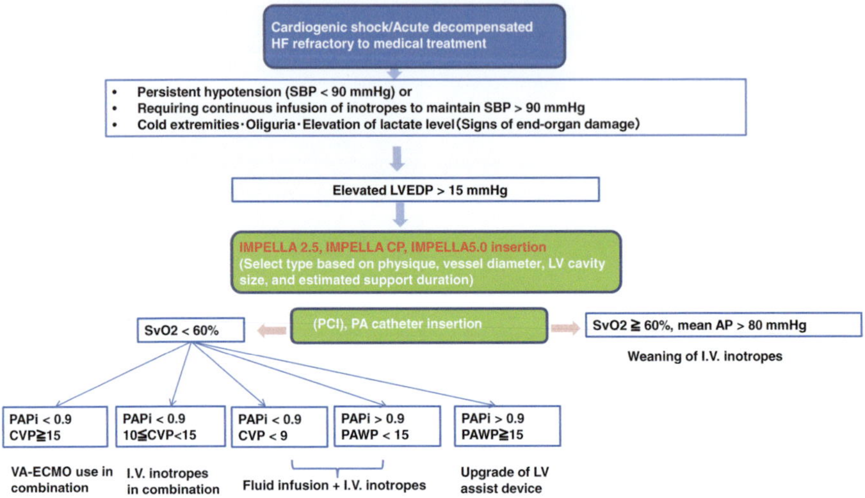

Fig. 7.4 Impella initiation and subsequent management

A suction alarm might be alerted if the inlet part contacts with the LV wall or any other structures and cannot vacuum sufficient blood. Pulmonary artery pulsatility index (PAPi) should be calculated to assess whether the suction alarm comes from right heart failure or from volume insufficiency. PAPi is calculated as follows: (systolic pulmonary artery pressure−diastolic pulmonary artery pressure)/(right atrial pressure). If PAPi is under 0.9, an additional approach to right ventricle (RV) failure should be considered, including administration of dobutamine, milrinone, or initiation of ECMO; Fig. 7.4). It is reported that the patient who achieved cardiac power output, calculated as (mean blood pressure × cardiac output)/451, >0.6 and lactate <4 mmol/L at 12–24 h after initiation of Impella support was associated with better survival [11].

7.6 Management of Hemolysis

Hemolysis occurs when strong share stress is added to the blood cells. For example, hemolysis may occur when a suction alarm sounds in addition to thrombus in the catheter or blood pump, or when a structure in the LV is adjacent to the inlet part, or the aortic valve or aortic wall is adjacent to the outlet part. If the color of urine changes to red, we should check urinary occult blood, serum level of LDH, creatinine, and indirect bilirubin. If hemolysis is highly suspected, we should perform echocardiography to see the device position, and the optimization of device position or patients' volume status is highly recommended. In many cases, hemolysis can be improved by lowering the support level (rotation speed) or increasing the volume status as well as the optimization of anticoagulant therapy. If hemolysis is not improved, free hemoglobin causes renal tubular dysfunction and acute kidney injury. In some cases, the administration of haptoglobin preparation might prevent the progression of renal injury.

7.7 Next Step from Impella

If patients are completely depending on the Impella support, next strategies should be considered, including the device upgrade from Impella 2.5 to Impella 5.0 or the bridge to the durable left ventricular assist device (LVAD), valvular intervention during the Impella support, or explanation of Impella, given patients' background and comorbidities.

In case of bridge to durable LVAD, patients should be listed to heart transplantation beforehand in Japan as of 2020. Given various tests that are required for the listing take several weeks, Impella would be converted to extracorporeal LVAD considering their durability. Of note, Impella 5.0, instead of Impella 2.5, can support approximately 1 month for the heart transplant listing and conversion to durable implantable LVAD (Fig. 7.2).

References

1. O'Neill WW, Schreiber T, Wohns DH, et al. The current use of Impella 2.5 in acute myocardial infarction complicated by cardiogenic shock: results from the USpella Registry. J Interv Cardiol. 2014;27:1–11.
2. Esposito ML, Zhang Y, Qiao X, et al. Left ventricular unloading before reperfusion promotes functional recovery after acute myocardial infarction. J Am Coll Cardiol. 2018;72:501–14.
3. Seyfarth M, Sibbing D, Bauer I, et al. A randomized clinical trial to evaluate the safety and efficacy of a percutaneous left ventricular assist device versus intra-aortic balloon pumping for treatment of cardiogenic shock caused by myocardial infarction. J Am Coll Cardiol. 2008;52:1584–8.
4. Ouweneel DM, Eriksen E, Sjauw KD, et al. Percutaneous mechanical circulatory support versus intra-aortic balloon pump in cardiogenic shock after acute myocardial infarction. J Am Coll Cardiol. 2017;69:278–87.
5. Batsides G, Massaro J, Cheung A, et al. Outcomes of Impella 5.0 in cardiogenic shock: a systematic review and meta-analysis. Innovations. 2018;13:254–60.
6. Hall SA, Uriel N, Carey SA, et al. Use of a percutaneous temporary circulatory support device as a bridge to decision during acute decompensation of advanced heart failure. J Heart Lung Transplant. 2018;37:100–6.
7. Schrage B, Ibrahim K, Loehn T, et al. Impella support for acute myocardial infarction complicated by cardiogenic shock. Circulation. 2019;139:1249–58.
8. Tschope C, Van Linthout S, Klein O, et al. Mechanical unloading by fulminant myocarditis: LV-IMPELLA, ECMELLA, BI-PELLA, and PROPELLA concepts. J Cardiovasc Transl Res. 2019;12:116–23.

9. Patel SM, Lipinski J, Al-Kindi SG, et al. Simultaneous venoarterial extracorporeal membrane oxygenation and percutaneous left ventricular decompression therapy with impella is associated with improved outcomes in refractory cardiogenic shock. ASAIO J. 2018;65(1):21–8.
10. Hasegawa-Tamba S, Sugi K, Gatate Y, et al. Successful bridge-to-recovery treatment in a young patient with fulminant eosinophilic myocarditis: roles of a percutaneous ventricular assist device and endomyocardial biopsy. Case Rep Emerg Med. 2019;2019:8236735.
11. Basir MB, Kapur NK, Patel K, et al. Improved outcomes associated with the use of shock protocols: updates from the National Cardiogenic Shock Initiative. Catheter Cardiovasc Interv. 2019;93:1173–83.

Chapter 8
MitraClip

Hiroshi Ueno and Koichiro Kinugawa

Abstract Patients with advanced heart failure often accompany severe functional mitral regurgitation refractory to optimal medical therapy. Surgical mitral valve repair or replacement might be effective in some of the cases, but it has been challenging particularly for the high-risk cases. Recently, percutaneous edge-to-edge mitral valve repair using the MitraClip system, which enables us to approach the mitral valve at relatively low risk, has been developed. Two prospective randomized control trials have drawn controversial results in terms of the clinical advantage of MitraClip system over the optimal medical therapy in patients with advanced heart failure and functional mitral regurgitation. Therefore, the clinical advantage of MitraClip system over the optimal medical therapy has not been fully established thus far. Nevertheless, given we often experience a significant improvement of such mitral regurgitation by using MitraClip system, optimal patient selection and management by the heart team might be a key to success.

Keywords Mitral regurgitation · Percutaneous intervention · Edge-to-edge repair

8.1 Introduction

Mitral regurgitation (MR) is the most frequent valvular disease [1]. Mitral valve consists of the complex of mitral annulus, leaflets, chords, papillary muscle, and left ventricular myocardium. MR is distinguished by two major causes: (1) degenerative MR including mitral valve prolapse and mitral chordal rupture and (2) functional MR resulting from the tethering of mitral valve due to left ventricular remodeling or the mitral annular enlargement (Fig. 8.1).

Given the prognosis of functional mitral regurgitation is worse when heart failure symptom develops, the early intervention to the mitral valve is highly recommended [2]. However, in the real-world practice, almost half of the patients with functional mitral regurgitation do not receive the surgery, given their high risk to receive the surgery due to high age, renal failure, and depressed cardiac function [3].

H. Ueno (✉) · K. Kinugawa
The Second Department of Internal Medicine, University of Toyama, Toyama, Japan

K. Kinugawa, T. Imamura (eds.), *Update of Non-Pharmacological Therapy for Heart Failure*, https://doi.org/10.1007/978-981-15-4843-7_8

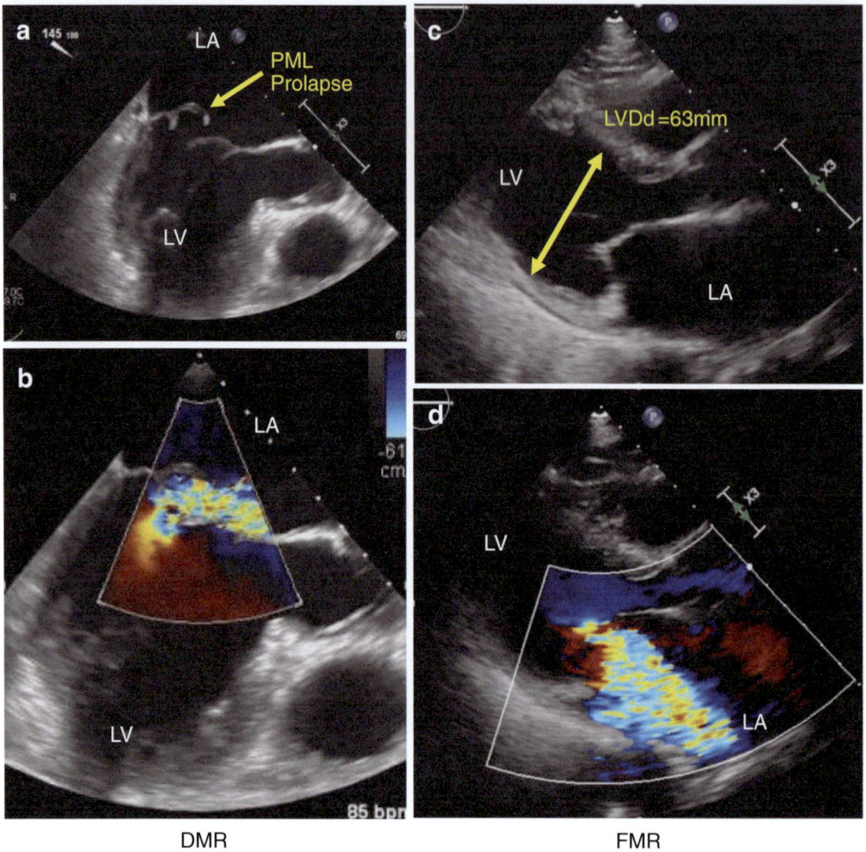

Fig. 8.1 Two mechanisms of mitral regurgitation (MR). (**a**) Left ventricular outflow tract (LVOT) view of transesophageal echo (TEE) reveals degenerative MR (DMR) due to posterior mitral valve leaflet (PML) prolapse. (**b**) Eccentric MR jet due to PML prolapse. (**c**) Parasternal long-axis view of transthoracic echo (TTE) reveals left ventricular dilation due to dilated cardiomyopathy (DCM). *LVDd* left ventricular end-diastolic dimension. (**d**) Concentric MR jet due to functional MR (FMR) caused by tethering

There has been no definite therapeutic strategy for such high-risk patients, except for optimal medical therapies, including beta-blocker, angiotensin converting enzyme inhibitor, mineralocorticoid receptor antagonist [4], or cardiac resynchronization therapy if applicable [5]. Surgical intervention has been considered for the patients' refractory to these medications. However, such a surgical intervention is assigned to Class IIb in the current guidelines, given the reduced cardiac function is high risk of perioperative comorbidities [5].

Considering that there is are lot of patients with advanced heart failure and MR refractory to surgical and medical approaches, a less invasive transcatheter intervention to the mitral valve has been innovated very recently.

8.2 Edge-to-Edge Repair (MitraClip®)

Surgical edge-to-edge technique in the mitral valve repair, introduced by a cardiac surgeon Alfieri in 1991 [6], and a transcatheter edge-to-edge repair of mitral valve, MitraClip (Abbott Vascular, Abbott Park, IL, USA), has been innovated in 1998.

Following the first-in-man study of MitraClip in 2003, a CE mark was obtained for the use of degenerative MR and functional MR in Europe in 2008 and the U.S. Food and Drug Administration approved MitraClip for the degenerative MR in 2013. In Japan, the MitraClip was approved for degenerative MR and functional MR under the insurance reimbursement in 2018. Given the favorable result of COAPT trial, the indication for the functional MR was also approved in the United States in 2018.

MitraClip system consists of a 24-Fr steerable guiding catheter (SGC) and a clip delivery system (CDS) with a clip located at the tip (Fig. 8.2). The CDS has two dials (medial-lateral direction and antero-posterior direction) to direct the clip toward the plane of mitral valve. The clip arm can be opened or closed by using the arm positioner knob attached to the CDS. You can try clipping repeatedly before releasing the clip from the CDS for the appropriate positioning.

The procedure is performed under the transesophageal echocardiography guide (Fig. 8.3). The CDS with a clip is delivered via the catheter on the origin of MR jet under transesophageal echocardiography guide, following the atrial septal puncture. The clip with its arm opened at 180° would be forwarded into the left ventricle at a right angle with the line of mitral valve. The CDS is lifted toward the valve with 120° of an arm angle until both leaflets sit on the arm, when both leaflets are clipped between the gripper and arm. After the confirmation of appropriate clipping by grading residual MR and valve stenosis, the clip is released from CDS.

Considering the degree of residual MR and mitral valve area, the indication of the second clip is discussed. Of note, the degree of MR might be underestimated due to reduced afterload of the left ventricle under the general anesthesia.

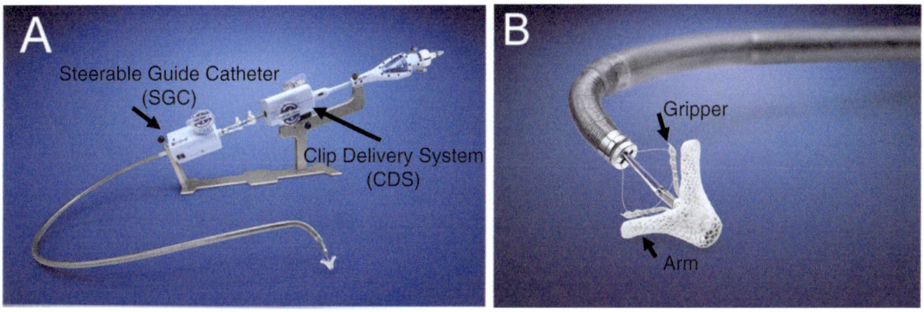

Source: Abbott Vascular

Fig. 8.2 (**a**) MitraClip system. (**b**) Clip of MitraClip NT

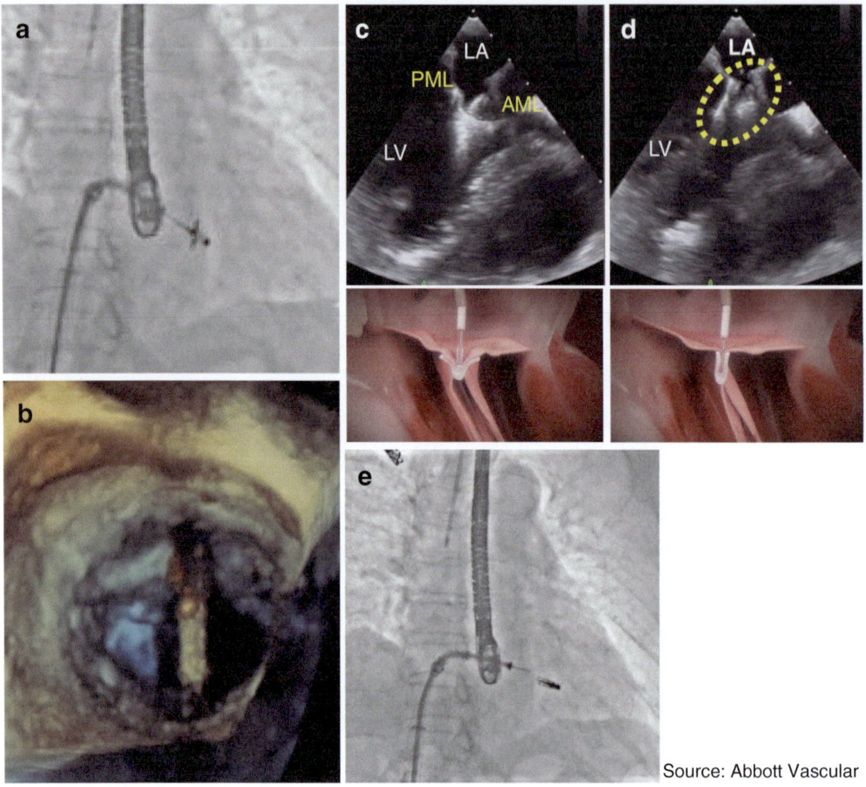

Fig. 8.3 (**a**) Fluoroscopic image of TEE-probe and MitraClip system. (**b**) Check the clip is orthogonal to the mitral valve leaflet from 3D-TEE surgeon's view. (**c**) The chip of anterior mitral valve leaflet (*AML*) and PML are on the clip arm. (**d**) The chip of AML and PML are grasping. (**e**) Fluoroscopic image after clip deployment

Vasoconstrictors might be considered to normalize afterload if necessary for the appropriate assessment of MR.

During the procedure, transesophageal echocardiography is a more useful tool to understand detailed anatomical device positioning than the fluoroscopic image. Echocardiologists and interventionists should collaborate with each other for the successful MitraClip procedure.

Following the procedure, approximately 8 mm of the idiopathic atrial septal defect remains, but most of them close gradually with a left to right shunt. If remained, transcatheter closure is considered [7]. For the hemostasis of the right femoral vein, a figure of eight technique with one suture is an easy and secure procedure [8].

Detailed indications of MitraClip for degenerative MR and functional MR would be discussed separately as follows. One of the most important tips is a detailed anatomical assessment of the mitral valve [9].

8.3 MitraClip® in Degenerative MR

Degenerative MR is a relatively common disease that develops in approximately 2% of the population [10]. The most major cause of degenerative MR is myxomatous degeneration, followed by chordal rupture, valvular prolapse, infectious endocarditis, and rheumatoid fever.

The gold standard is surgical interventions including mitral valve repair or replacement, and the repair is recommended for its superiority in the long-term outcome [11]. However, approximately half of the patients are not actually indicated for the surgery, given high age, renal dysfunction, and a history of open heart surgery [12]. Mehta and colleagues reported 17% mortality and 36% morbidity in patients aged over 80 years who received mitral valve surgery [13].

MitraClip procedure, a less invasive transcatheter edge-to-edge mitral valve clipping, was innovated for such high-risk populations. Thus far, many studies have demonstrated the safety and efficacy of the MitraClip procedure. Of note, Endovascular Valve Edge-to-Edge Repair Study II (EVEREST II) is the sole prospective multicenter randomized trial that compared MitraClip procedure with conventional surgical intervention [14]. In this study, 279 patients with symptomatic MR were randomized into the MitraClip arm and the surgical arm (repair or replacement) as a proportion of 2:1. Of them, 73% was degenerative MR, and those with reduced cardiac function (left ventricular end-diastolic diameter over 55 mm or left ventricular ejection fraction below 25%) were excluded. The rate of recurrence of MR requiring reoperation was higher in the MitraClip arm over the surgical arm (20 vs. 2%), whereas 1-year and 4-year severity of MR and mortality were statistically comparable between the arms. Major adverse events were also statistically not different between the two arms except for the lower incidence of transfusion in the MitraClip arm (13 vs. 45%).

EVEREST High-Risk Registry, a sub-analysis of EVEREST II trial [15], assessed 78 patients with estimated survival ≥12% who received MitraClip procedure or medical therapy. One-year survival was superior in the MitraClip group compared with the medical group (76 vs. 55%) as well as the lower 1-year rate of heart failure recurrence in the MitraClip group (16 vs. 42%).

In the REALIS trial which included 127 inoperable patients with degenerative MR, MitraClip procedure suppressed a 1-year heart failure readmission rate in 73%. Given those with residual MR ≤2° had over 80% of freedom from the events, residual MR ≤2 is set as an acute success of MitraClip procedure [16].

Given these results, the surgical intervention is recommended as a first choice for the severe degenerative MR, followed by the second choice MitraClip procedure for the high-risk or inoperable cases. The AHA/ACC guidelines recommend MitraClip procedure for those with symptomatic severe degenerative MR who have a reasonable life expectancy but a prohibitive surgical risk because of severe comorbidities (Class IIb) [17]. ESC/EACTS guidelines also recommend MitraClip procedure in patients with symptomatic severe degenerative MR who fulfill the echocardiographic criteria of eligibility and are judged inoperable or at high surgical risk (Class IIb) [5].

In Japan, although there is no recommendation in any guidelines, an appropriate use principle is proposed, which states that MitraClip should be considered in patients with symptomatic severe inoperable MR refractory to guideline-directed medical therapy, which has suitable anatomy for the procedure and a probability to improve MR and heart failure symptom.

8.4 MitraClip® in Functional MR

Functional MR develops in patients without any structural disorders. Instead, the dominant etiologies of functional MR are left ventricular remodeling due to cardiomyopathy and atrial remodeling due to long-term atrial fibrillation. In patients with left ventricular dilatation, the tethering of mitral leaflets is the dominant cause of "classical" functional MR. In patients with atrial remodeling, the worsening of coaptation of mitral leaflets due to the enlargement of the left atrium is the dominant cause of "atrial" functional MR [18].

Guideline-directed medical therapy is considered to treat background heart failure. However, the implication of such medications in improving functional MR remains suspicious [19]. Cardiac resynchronization therapy is also considered in patients with functional MR, but the clinical implication remains unknown. Surgical intervention to the mitral valve is also considered. Its improvement in left ventricular remodeling and heart failure symptoms has been demonstrated, whereas the survival benefit of the surgical intervention remains undemonstrated [20]. Therefore, AHA/ACC and ESC/EACTS guidelines recommend surgical intervention to the mitral valve alone as class IIb. Furthermore, half of the patients with functional MR cannot receive guideline-directed surgical intervention given their reduced cardiac function [3].

MitraClip procedure has several advantages, including: (1) it can be performed via venous approach; (2) real-time assessment of MR during the repair can be observed; (3) clipping can be tried multiple times; and (4) the procedure does not require contrast medium.

A sub-analysis of the EVEREST II High Risk Cohort was reported to show the clinical outcome of MitraClip procedure on the functional MR [21]. Patients with moderate or greater MR who had STS score above 12% or high risk for the surgery received MitraClip procedure. Of them, 246/351 had functional MR. At discharge, 88% had mild or less MR, and 30-day mortality was 4.1%. At 12 months, the prevalence of mild or less MR, left ventricular diameter, NYHA functional class were all superior to pre-procedural conditions.

Following the report, prospective randomized control trials comparing guideline-directed medical therapy arm versus MitraClip add-on arm were conducted to investigate the prognostic implication of MitraClip on the functional MR. Currently, MITRA-FR trial [22] and COAPT trial [23] have been reported.

In the MITRA-FR trial, 304 patients with functional MR who had left ventricular ejection fraction 15–40%, regurgitant fraction ≥30 mL, and NYHA functional class

II–IV were randomized into 152 medical arm and 152 MitraClip add-on arm. During the MitraClip procedure, cardiovascular complications developed in five patients and cardiac tamponade happened in two patients. At 12 months, there was no statistically significant difference in the primary composite endpoint, i.e., all-cause death and unplanned rehospitalization for heart failure.

In the COAPT trial, 614 patients with functional MR who had left ventricular ejection fraction 25–50% (31.3 ± 9.3% on average), moderate or severe regurgitation, and NYHA functional class II–IV were randomized into 312 medical arm and 302 MitraClip add-on arm. Of all, 60% had ischemic etiology. The MitraClip add-on arm had a lower 24-month heart failure readmission rate compared with the medical arm (38.5 vs. 67.9%, $p < 0.001$). All-cause mortality during the 24-month observational period was also significantly lower in the MitraClip add-on arm compared to the medical arm (29.1 vs. 46.1%, $p < 0.001$) (Fig. 8.4).

There are several discussions to explain discrepancy between the two studies [24]: (1) doubled sample size; (2) difference in the observational period (1 year vs. 2 years); (3) MITRA-FR trial had more enlarged left ventricle (135 ± 35 vs. 101 ± 34 mL/m^2) and reduced left ventricular ejection fraction (15–40 vs. 20–50%) compared with the COAPT trial; and (4) the degree of MR was lower in the

a

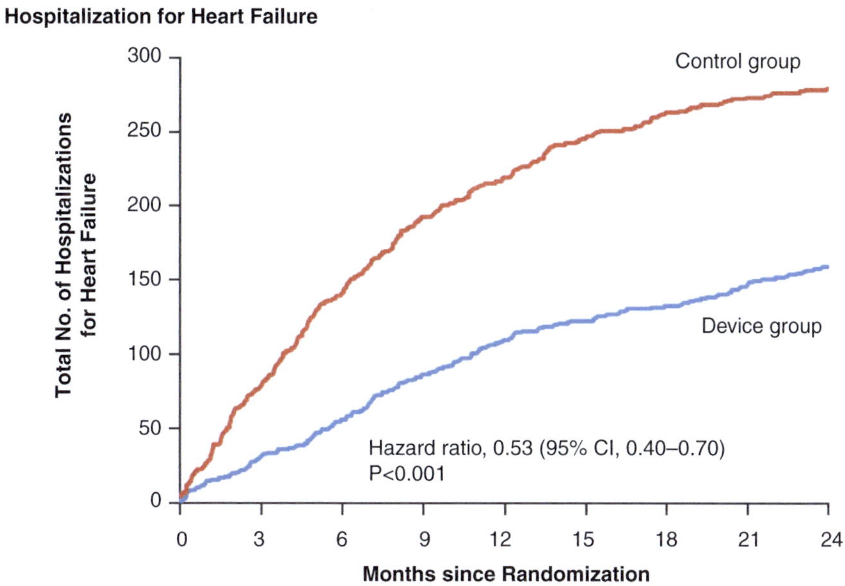

No. at Risk									
Control group	312	294	271	245	219	176	145	121	88
Device group	302	286	269	253	236	191	178	161	124

Fig. 8.4 (**a**) MitraClip with guideline-directed medical therapy (GDMT) reduced significantly hospitalizations for heart failure than GDMT only in the COAPT trial. (**b**) MitraClip with GDMT reduced all-cause mortality over 36 months than GDMT only in the COAPT trial

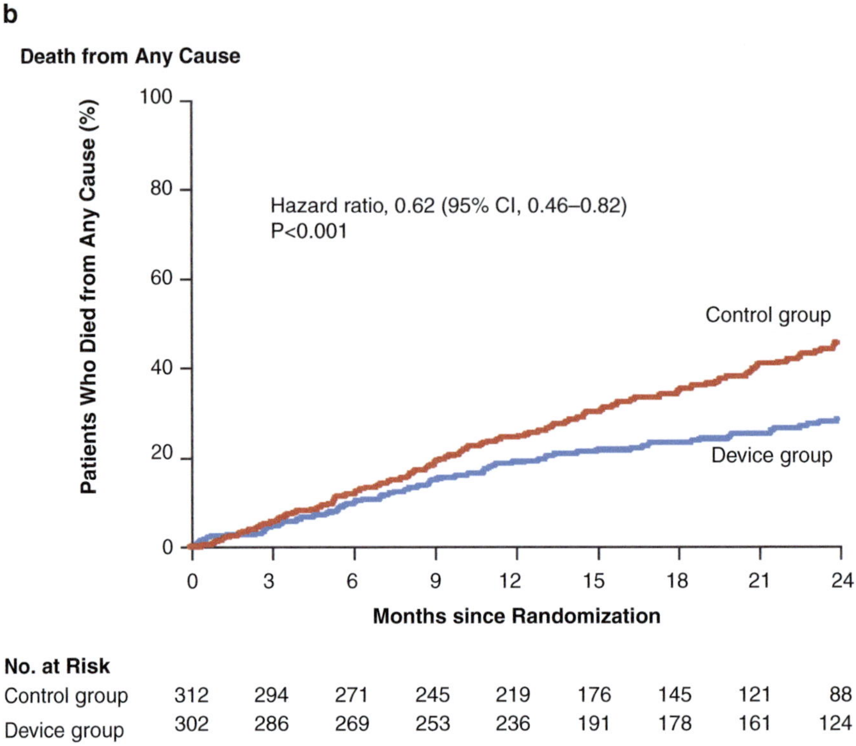

Fig. 8.4 (continued)

MITRA-FR trial than the COAPT trial (effective regurgitant orifice area, 31 ± 10 vs. 41 ± 15 mm^2). Given these differences, left ventricular function was a dominant prognostic factor in the MITRA-FR trial, whereas MR itself was a dominant prognostic factor in the COAPT trial. In other words, the impact of MitraClip might be more dominant in the COAPT trial than the MITRA-FR trial. Furthermore, the protocol of medication was different between the two trials: medications were sufficiently optimized at baseline in the COAPT trial, whereas not sufficiently optimized in the MITRA-FR trial.

Currently, the indication of MitraClip in patients with functional MR is (1) symptomatic MR refractory to guideline-directed medical therapy, (2) high operative risk, (3) left ventricular ejection fraction above 20%, (4) moderate or greater MR, and (5) anatomical feature applicable to the procedure [5]. Considering the current evidence, an algorithm to consider intervention to the functional MR in patients with reduced left ventricular ejection fraction might be proposed (Fig. 8.5) [5].

More evidence should be accumulated based on these trials to expand the indication of the MitraClip procedure. Next concerns would be intervention to the mitral annulus and tricuspid regurgitation that often develops secondary to the MR.

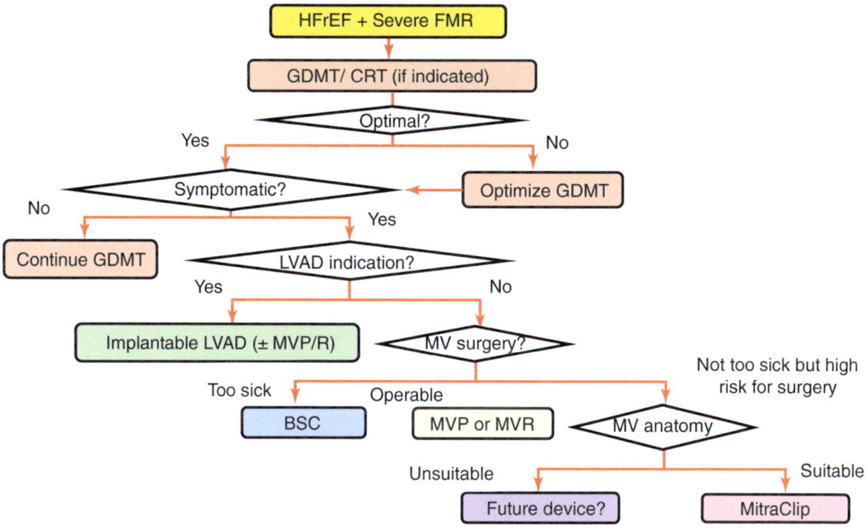

Fig. 8.5 Treatment algorithm in patients with reduced left ventricular ejection fraction and functional MR. *HFrEF* heart failure with reduced ejection fraction, *FMR* functional mitral regurgitation, *GDMT* guideline-directed medical therapy, *CRT* cardiac resynchronization therapy, *LVAD* left ventricular assist device, *BSC* best supportive care, *MVP* mitral valve plasty, *MVR* mitral valve replacement

Acknowledgment

Conflicts of Interest None

References

1. Nkomo VT, Gardin JM, Skelton TN, Gottdiener JS, Scott CG, Enriquez-Sarano M. Burden of valvular heart diseases: a population-based study. Lancet. 2006;368(9540):1005–11.
2. Ling LH, Enriquez-Sarano M, Seward JB, Tajik AJ, Schaff HV, Bailey KR, et al. Clinical outcome of mitral regurgitation due to flail leaflet. N Engl J Med. 1996;335(19):1417–23.
3. Mirabel M, Iung B, Baron G, Messika-Zeitoun D, Detaint D, Vanoverschelde JL, et al. What are the characteristics of patients with severe, symptomatic, mitral regurgitation who are denied surgery? Eur Heart J. 2007;28(11):1358–65.
4. Ponikowski P, Voors AA, Anker SD, Bueno H, Cleland JGF, Coats AJS, et al. 2016 ESC guidelines for the diagnosis and treatment of acute and chronic heart failure: the task force for the diagnosis and treatment of acute and chronic heart failure of the European Society of Cardiology (ESC) developed with the special contribution of the heart failure association (HFA) of the ESC. Eur Heart J. 2016;37(27):2129–200.
5. Baumgartner H, Falk V, Bax JJ, De Bonis M, Hamm C, Holm PJ, et al. 2017 ESC/EACTS guidelines for the management of valvular heart disease. Eur Heart J. 2017;38(36):2739–91.
6. Alfieri O, Maisano F, De Bonis M, Stefano PL, Torracca L, Oppizzi M, et al. The double-orifice technique in mitral valve repair: a simple solution for complex problems. J Thorac Cardiovasc Surg. 2001;122(4):674–81.

7. Beri N, Singh GD, Smith TW, Fan D, Boyd WD, Rogers JH. Iatrogenic atrial septal defect closure after transseptal mitral valve interventions: indications and outcomes. Catheter Cardiovasc Interv. 2019;94(6):829–36.
8. Cilingiroglu M, Salinger M, Zhao D, Feldman T. Technique of temporary subcutaneous "figure-of-eight" sutures to achieve hemostasis after removal of large-caliber femoral venous sheaths. Catheter Cardiovasc Interv. 2011;78(1):155–60.
9. Taramasso M, Gavazzoni M, Nickenig G, Maisano F. Transcatheter mitral repair and replacement: which procedure for which patient? EuroIntervention. 2019;15(10):867–74.
10. Enriquez-Sarano M, Akins CW, Vahanian A. Mitral regurgitation. Lancet. 2009;373(9672):1382–94.
11. Suri RM, Schaff HV, Dearani JA, Sundt TM 3rd, Daly RC, Mullany CJ, et al. Survival advantage and improved durability of mitral repair for leaflet prolapse subsets in the current era. Ann Thorac Surg. 2006;82(3):819–26.
12. Bach DS, Awais M, Gurm HS, Kohnstamm S. Failure of guideline adherence for intervention in patients with severe mitral regurgitation. J Am Coll Cardiol. 2009;54(9):860–5.
13. Mehta RH, Eagle KA, Coombs LP, Peterson ED, Edwards FH, Pagani FD, et al. Influence of age on outcomes in patients undergoing mitral valve replacement. Ann Thorac Surg. 2002;74(5):1459–67.
14. Feldman T, Foster E, Glower DD, Kar S, Rinaldi MJ, Fail PS, et al. Percutaneous repair or surgery for mitral regurgitation. N Engl J Med. 2011;364(15):1395–406.
15. Whitlow PL, Feldman T, Pedersen WR, Lim DS, Kipperman R, Smalling R, et al. Acute and 12-month results with catheter-based mitral valve leaflet repair: the EVEREST II (endovascular valve edge-to-edge repair) high risk study. J Am Coll Cardiol. 2012;59(2):130–9.
16. Lim DS, Reynolds MR, Feldman T, Kar S, Herrmann HC, Wang A, et al. Improved functional status and quality of life in prohibitive surgical risk patients with degenerative mitral regurgitation after transcatheter mitral valve repair. J Am Coll Cardiol. 2014;64(2):182–92.
17. Nishimura RA, Otto CM, Bonow RO, Carabello BA, Erwin JP 3rd, Guyton RA, et al. 2014 AHA/ACC guideline for the management of patients with valvular heart disease: a report of the American College of Cardiology/American Heart Association task force on practice guidelines. J Am Coll Cardiol. 2014;63(22):e57–185.
18. Ring L, Dutka DP, Wells FC, Fynn SP, Shapiro LM, Rana BS. Mechanisms of atrial mitral regurgitation: insights using 3D transoesophageal echo. Eur Heart J Cardiovasc Imaging. 2014;15(5):500–8.
19. Agricola E, Ielasi A, Oppizzi M, Faggiano P, Ferri L, Calabrese A, et al. Long-term prognosis of medically treated patients with functional mitral regurgitation and left ventricular dysfunction. Eur J Heart Fail. 2009;11(6):581–7.
20. Mihaljevic T, Lam BK, Rajeswaran J, Takagaki M, Lauer MS, Gillinov AM, et al. Impact of mitral valve annuloplasty combined with revascularization in patients with functional ischemic mitral regurgitation. J Am Coll Cardiol. 2007;49(22):2191–201.
21. Glower DD, Kar S, Trento A, Lim DS, Bajwa T, Quesada R, et al. Percutaneous mitral valve repair for mitral regurgitation in high-risk patients: results of the EVEREST II study. J Am Coll Cardiol. 2014;64(2):172–81.
22. Obadia JF, Messika-Zeitoun D, Leurent G, Iung B, Bonnet G, Piriou N, et al. Percutaneous repair or medical treatment for secondary mitral regurgitation. N Engl J Med. 2018;379(24):2297–306.
23. Stone GW, Lindenfeld J, Abraham WT, Kar S, Lim DS, Mishell JM, et al. Transcatheter mitral-valve repair in patients with heart failure. N Engl J Med. 2018;379(24):2307–18.
24. Pibarot P, Delgado V, Bax JJ. MITRA-FR vs. COAPT: lessons from two trials with diametrically opposed results. Eur Heart J Cardiovasc Imaging. 2019;20(6):620–4.

Chapter 9
MVP/LV Plasty

Akira Shiose and Satoshi Kimura

Abstract Heart failure is one of the most important health problems in the world. Ironically, advancements in medical therapy have resulted in an increasing number of patients who are living with severe left ventricular dysfunction and congestive heart failure. There are several non-pharmacological therapies for heart failure. At present, heart transplantation is a definitive therapy of congestive heart failure. However, this procedure can be offered to limited patients for the shortage of organ donors. Therefore, alternative surgical therapies such as partial left ventriculectomy, mitral valve plasty, and left ventriculoplasty have been introduced for the treatment of congestive heart failure. Surgeons must refine surgical indications for determining which patients are the best candidates for each of these procedures.

Keyword Partial left ventriculectomy · Mitral valve plasty · Left ventriculoplasty · Endoventricular circular patch plasty · Septal anterior ventricular exclusion

9.1 Introduction

Heart failure (HF) is an often-encountered common disease in the elderly, and one of the refractory and life-threatening, progressive, malignant diseases. HF has been the leading cause of morbidity and mortality in developed countries. In addition, it needs frequent hospitalization and a great deal of cost. As aging of the population is advancing, the incidence of HF is increasing even more. The ultimate treatment for end-stage HF is currently cardiac transplantation. On the ground of an absolute shortage of organ donors, however, this treatment is available to limited patients only. Most transplant candidates have to be still waiting for a suitable donor organ for a long time. Whereas sophisticated medical therapies can sometimes improve patient's condition, it cannot always prevent deterioration of ventricular dysfunction. Therefore, surgical options such as partial left ventriculectomy (PLV), mitral valve plasty (MVP), and left ventriculoplasty (LV plasty) are important for the treatment of congestive HF.

A. Shiose (✉) · S. Kimura
Department of Cardiovascular Surgery, Kyushu University, Fukuoka, Japan
e-mail: shiose@heart.med.kyushu-u.ac.jp

K. Kinugawa, T. Imamura (eds.), *Update of Non-Pharmacological Therapy for Heart Failure*, https://doi.org/10.1007/978-981-15-4843-7_9

9.2 Partial Left Ventriculectomy

Surgical ventricular plasty have been originally developed for ischemic cardiomyopathy (ICM). PLV was introduced for the aim of the improvement of left ventricular contractility by reducing left ventricular volume with partial resection of the posterior wall of the left ventricle (LV) by Batista in 1996 [1]. Since then, this method has rapidly spread worldwide as so-called Batista's surgery. This procedure was anticipated to improve left ventricular function with decrease of myocardial oxygen consumption by reducing pressure and tension on the left ventricular wall in accordance of Laplace's law.

9.2.1 Surgical Procedure

Under cardioplegic arrest with ordinary cardiopulmonary bypass support, an incision is made at the apex of the LV and is extended toward the base. The cavity of the LV is inspected, and LV volume reduction is achieved by resecting LV muscle between the papillary muscles with care to avoid injuring the left circumflex artery. The left ventriculectomy is then closed with a double layer of monofilament sutures for hemostasis (Fig. 9.1).

MVP or mitral valve replacement (MVR) is usually performed concomitantly with PLV to ensure against mitral valve prolapse and insufficiency. After the inspection of the left ventricular cavity, the distance between the anterior and posterior papillary muscles is determined. If the heart is massively enlarged, excision of the papillary muscles and MVR may be necessary to achieve satisfactory anatomic dimensions. Also, mitral valve annuloplasty and valvuloplasty may be performed if the valve is degenerated. These procedures can be done through the left ventricular incision.

9.2.2 Outcomes

The concept of surgical size reduction of the nonischemic dilated LV is similar to that used in ICM. However, the difference from the surgical treatment of ICM is that remaining viable cardiac muscle with deteriorated function is removed instead of infarcted region in ICM patients. Therefore, outcomes were variable owing to nonspecific exclusion of the lateral wall, which might have contained remaining viable muscle [2, 3].

Batista et al. reported that PLV was conducted in 120 patients with end-stage nonischemic dilated cardiomyopathy (NIDCM), most of which were New York Heart Association (NYHA) class IV. The procedure consisted of wedge resection of LV muscle from the apex to the base of the heart. Depending on the distance between

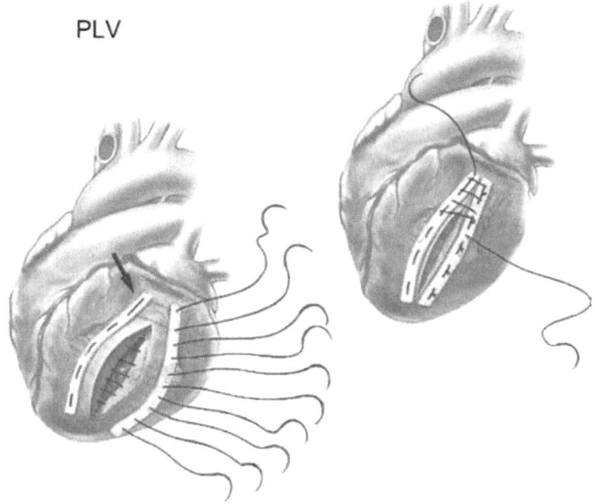

Fig. 9.1 Partial left ventriculectomy (PLV) procedure with excision of the lateral ventricular wall, and ventricular closure with wide mattress sutures to restore an elliptical form (adapted with permission from Suma et al. [2])

both papillary muscles, the mitral valve apparatus was either preserved, repaired, or replaced with bioprosthesis. The 30-day mortality was about 20% and the 2-year survival was almost half. Although 10% of surviving patients showed no improvement in NYHA class, most of the survivors improved their symptoms. They concluded that PLV can be used to treat end-stage NIDCM and further studies and a longer follow-up are necessitated [4]. After this report, additional tests were conducted. The Cleveland Clinic prospectively evaluated this procedure for patients of NYHA class III or IV heart transplant candidates with LV end-diastolic diameter >70 mm. As a result, survival was 80% and 60% at 1 and 3 years after surgery and freedom from failure, including implantation of left ventricular assist device, return to class IV HF, relisting for transplantation, and death, was 49% and 26%, respectively, which were considered low [5]. Although the symptom and LV function certainly improved in some patients over time, it was difficult to predict preoperatively which patient received the beneficial effect with PLV. It is unclear and restricted of the efficiency of PLV to nonischemic cardiomyopathy. Therefore, ACCF/AHA guideline for the management of HF provides the recommendation class III since 2013 [6]. In view of its uncertain beneficial effect, it may be appropriate to try PLV procedure in restricted situations that transplantation is not indicated or as a biological bridge to transplantation.

9.3 Mitral Valve Plasty

It is acceptable that durable and reliable MVP is an effective procedure for degenerative mitral valve regurgitation (MR) compared to mitral valve replacement (MVR). However, surgical strategies for secondary MR with ICM and nonischemic cardiomyopathy are controversial.

Secondary MR is common in patients with HF and adversely affects survival and quality of life [7]. The etiology is complex and multifactorial, characterized by LV dilatation and dysfunction or mitral annulus dilatation, while mitral valve itself is structurally intact. LV dilatation causes papillary muscle displacement and leaflet tethering, leading to incomplete valve closure and regurgitation. LV dysfunction with reduced LV contractility results in reduced valve closing forces, leading to regurgitation. Mitral annulus dilatation can occur due to LV or left atrial dilatation resulting in atrial fibrillation. Once it is established, secondary MR accelerates the progression of ventricular remodeling that increases the severity of MR and congestive HF [8]. The surgical management of patients with secondary MR is challenging and controversial at times. The goals of treatment of secondary MR are to restore the competence of the mitral valve and to stop or reverse ventricular remodeling.

9.3.1 Restrictive Mitral Annuloplasty

Restrictive mitral annuloplasty is currently the most common surgical procedure of secondary MR. It is usually performed with a complete and rigid ring. The ring must be at least one or two sizes smaller than the size necessary to improve leaflet coaptation [9]. Complete restrictive mitral annuloplasty with undersized complete rigid ring to improve leaflet coaptation is the most widely applied technique [10, 11]. However, restrictive mitral annuloplasty is associated with high rates of MR recurrence because of primarily addressing only annular dilatation and not LV. In addition, it can increase posterior mitral leaflet tethering when there is a mismatch between ring size and LV dimension [12].

9.3.2 Subvalvular Procedures

Therefore, additional subvalvular procedures, such as secondary chordal cutting [13], relocation of the displaced posterior papillary muscle with a transventricular suture [14], and papillary muscle repositioning with a transventricular suture [15, 16], have been proposed to overcome posterior leaflet tethering. Reports on subvalvular repair techniques are limited by small sample size and single-center, retrospective designs. Papillary muscle approximation in addition to complete surgical myocardial revascularization and undersized restrictive mitral annuloplasty exerted a long-term beneficial effect on LV remodeling and more effectively restored the mitral valve geometric configuration in secondary MR, which improved long-term cardiac outcomes, but did not produce differences in overall mortality and quality of life in a randomized trial [17].

The impact of MVP on mortality and recurrence in secondary MR is unclear and MVR was recently recommended rather than MVP [18].

9.3.3 *Guidelines for Mitral Valve Surgery in Secondary MR*

2014 AHA/ACC valvular heart disease guidelines suggest that mitral valve surgery is reasonable for patients with chronic severe secondary MR undergoing coronary artery bypass grafting (CABG) or aortic valve replacement (Class IIa) and mitral valve surgery may be considered for severely symptomatic patients with chronic severe secondary MR who have persistent symptoms despite optimal guideline-directed medical therapy (GDMT) for HF (Class IIb) [19]. Newest AHA/ACC updated guidelines updated two new and modified recommendations in 2017 [20]. The added state is that chordal-sparing MVR over MVP is reasonable if operation is considered for severely symptomatic patients with chronic severe ischemic MR and persistent symptoms despite GDMT for HF. A randomized control trial (RCT) has shown that MVP is associated with a higher rate of recurrence of moderate or severe MR than that associated with MVR in patients with severe, symptomatic, ischemic MR, with no difference in mortality rate at 2 years' follow-up [21]. Another modified state is that the usefulness of MVP is uncertain in patients with chronic, moderate, ischemic MR undergoing CABG. Although 2014 guideline recommended the superiority of MVP in this group of patients, RCTs showed no clinical benefit of MVP with increased risk of postoperative complications [18, 22].

9.4 Left Ventriculoplasty for the Treatment of Ischemic Cardiomyopathy

Left ventricular aneurysmectomy to treat extensive dyskinetic area resulting from transmural myocardial infarction was first performed by Cooley in 1958 [23–25]. There has been ever reported the effectiveness of this method. Left ventriculoplasty (LV plasty) was also believed to improve cardiac function, in the same manner as the treatment of left ventricular aneurysm. Because of the spread of early intervention in the treatment of acute myocardial infarction, the number of patients with persistent akinesis due to subendocardial infarction tends to be higher than dyskinesis due to transmural infarction. However, after a relatively extensive myocardial infarction, and regardless of whether the infarcted region shows dyskinesis or akinesis, LV remodeling occurs, causing a gradual expansion of the non-infarcted region along with deteriorated function. This pathogenesis ultimately leads to ICM, namely, the decrease of contractility of entire LV. In such cases, LV plasty is applied with the aim to improve both contractility of the remaining non-infarcted region and LV dilatation and morphological changes caused by the reshaping during surgical resection or plasty of the infarcted region.

9.4.1 Surgical Procedure

9.4.1.1 Endoventricular Circular Patch Plasty

Dor et al. first described the technique of endoventricular circular patch plasty (EVCPP), which is used to treat patients with post-infarcted left ventricular scar [26]. EVCPP is performed with cardioplegic heart arrest. The LV is opened in the center of the anterior lesion. In akinetic segments, the junction between scarred and normal muscle is not as clearly defined as in dyskinetic aneurysms. An endoventricular circular suture, so-called Fontan stitch, is placed to restore the "neck" of the contracting ventricle, thereby providing a more normal oval curvature of the LV. The circular suture is passed in the fibrous tissue above the transitional zone between normal and scarred tissue, followed by closure with an approximately 3 × 4 cm Dacron patch (Fig. 9.2). After closure, the excluded external tissue is folded to reinforce the suture line. With this procedure, the LV is thus restored at an anteroseptal site with a small patch.

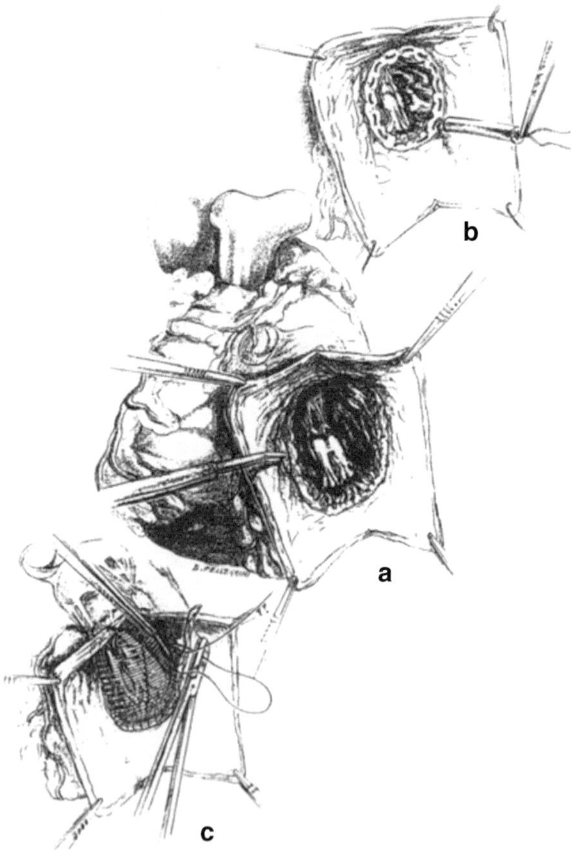

Fig. 9.2 (**a**) Aspect of the LV cavity after endocardial resection. (**b**) Endoventricular continuous suture to shorten the opening (Fontan stitch). (**c**) Dacron patch closure with or without pericardial strips (adapted with permission from Dor et al. [27])

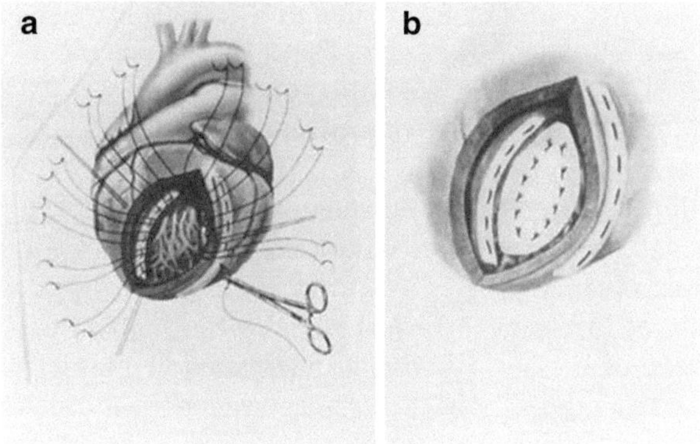

Fig. 9.3 (**a**) The LV is longitudinally incised anteriorly, and is thoroughly investigated by endocardial inspection and by palpation of the beating ventricular wall to detect the extension of the akinetic area. Endocardial interrupted mattress sutures with Teflon strip are placed along the posterior septum. The anterior free wall is excluded by placing trans-myocardial interrupted mattress sutures with Teflon strip. (**b**) These mattress stitches are sutured to the Dacron patch in a longitudinal oval shape (usually 1 cm width and 3–4 cm length) (adapted with permission from Suma et al. [2])

9.4.1.2 Septal Anterior Ventricular Exclusion

In addition, the surgical technique known as septal anterior ventricular exclusion (SAVE), in which a vertical patch is sewn at the border between the infarcted area and healthy regions, has also been performed [28]. SAVE operation is usually performed on the beating heart under cardiopulmonary bypass support. The LV is opened from the apex to the base along the left anterior descending artery. While kinesis of the LV wall is examined by preoperative examination, palpation of the LV muscle during its contraction allows differentiation between akinetic and normal muscle. Multiple mattress stitches are placed along the exclusion line of the septum, with direction that proceeds from the apex to septal myocardial infarction region. Dacron patch is trimmed to create a longitudinal shape, approximately 3 × 8 cm, and is placed along the site of the exclusion with sutures. The external tissue is closed with running sutures for hemostasis (Fig. 9.3). In this technique, Fontan stitch is not required to ensure that the LV has a shortened transverse diameter and an oval shape.

Both LV plasty methods allow for the LV volume reduction and make it possible to ensure that the morphology of the LV returns to its original oval shape.

9.4.2 Indications and Outcomes

The preoperative LV end-systolic volume index (LVESVI) of >100 mL/m^2 was demonstrated to be an independent predictor of long-term mortality following isolated CABG [29]. Therefore, LV plasty has been concomitantly performed in patients with dilated LV due to ICM [30]. LV plasty reduced late mortality and morbidity compared with CABG alone in patients with large LV [31]. Dor et al. concluded that EVCPP associated with CABG provides surviving patients with significantly improved cardiac function in patients with either a large akinetic or dyskinetic scar and severe LV dysfunction [26]. Late results were improved in the overall population, but a higher late mortality rate was observed in ICM patients with a larger preoperative LV and leaving a larger postoperative LV [30].

On the basis of long-term experiences, following criteria are suggested for EVCPP, in patients of any age: anteroseptal infarction and dilated LV (end-diastolic volume index >100 mL/m^2), and depressed ejection fraction (<20%), and LV regional asynergy (either dyskinesia or akinesia) >35% of the ventricular perimeter, and symptoms of angina, HF, arrhythmias, or inducible ischemia on provocative tests in asymptomatic patients. On the contrary, severe pulmonary artery pressure >60 mmHg, and severe right ventricular dysfunction, and regional asynergy without LV dilatation associated with risk of too small a residual chamber are considered relative contraindication [32].

Another LV plasty technique, SAVE, is easy to reshape dilated LV from spherical to ellipsoid form, and resultant improved configuration may contribute to overall results [33]. On the other hand, LV compliance was significantly reduced immediately after the operation and was not improved thereafter [34]. These findings, progression LV sphericity after EVCPP and reduced LV compliance after SAVE, seem to be related the problem of the procedure itself.

The Surgical Treatment for Ischemic Heart Failure (STICH) trial was a randomized trial, designed to define the role of cardiac surgery in the treatment of patients with ICM. Adding LV plasty to CABG reduced the LV volume, as compared with CABG alone. However, no significant difference was observed in the primary outcome including any cause of death and cardiac cause of hospitalization [35]. Therefore, it has been unclear whether LV volume reduction acquired with LV plasty causes negative remodeling. Surgeons have to know the operative technique off course. In addition, they must determine the LV function and the volume and size before and after LV plasty.

References

1. Batista RJV, Santos JLV, Takeshita N, Bocchino L, Lima PN, Cunha MA. Partial left ventriculectomy to improve left ventricular function in end-stage heart disease. J Card Surg. 1996;11(2):96–7.
2. Suma H, Isomura T, Horii T, Buckberg G. Role of site selection for left ventriculoplasty to treat idiopathic dilated cardiomyopathy. Heart Fail Rev. 2005;9(4):329–36.
3. Ascione R, Lim KHH, Chamberlain M, Al-Ruzzeh S, Angelini GD. Early and late results of partial left ventriculectomy: single center experience and review of the literature. J Card Surg. 2003;18(3):190–6.
4. Batista RJV, Verde J, Nery P, Bocchino L, Takeshita N, Bhayana JN, et al. Partial left ventriculectomy to treat end-stage heart disease. Ann Thorac Surg. 1997;64(3):634–8.

5. Franco-Cereceda A, McCarthy PM, Blackstone EH, Hoercher KJ, White JA, Young JB, et al. Partial left ventriculectomy for dilated cardiomyopathy: is this an alternative to transplantation? J Thorac Cardiovasc Surg. 2001;121(5):879–93.
6. Yancy CW, Jessup M, Bozkurt B, Butler J, Casey DE, Drazner MH, et al. 2013 ACCF/AHA guideline for the management of heart failure. Circulation. 2013;128:e240–327.
7. Goliasch G, Bartko PE, Pavo N, Neuhold S, Wurm R, Mascherbauer J, et al. Refining the prognostic impact of functional mitral regurgitation in chronic heart failure. Eur Heart J. 2018;39(1):39–46.
8. Lancellotti P, Marwick T, Pierard LA. How to manage ischaemic mitral regurgitation. Heart. 2008;94(11):1497–502.
9. Spoor MT, Geltz A, Bolling SF. Flexible versus nonflexible mitral valve rings for congestive heart failure: differential durability of repair. Circulation. 2006;114(Suppl 1):67–71.
10. Asgar AW, Mack MJ, Stone GW. Secondary mitral regurgitation in heart failure. J Am Coll Cardiol. 2015;65(12):1231–48.
11. Baumgartner H, Falk V, Bax JJ, De Bonis M, Hamm C, Holm PJ, et al. ESC/EACTS guidelines for the management of valvular heart disease. Eur Heart J. 2017;38:2739–91.
12. Capoulade R, Zeng X, Overbey JR, Ailawadi G, Alexander JH, Ascheim D, et al. Impact of left ventricular to mitral valve ring mismatch on recurrent ischemic mitral regurgitation after ring annuloplasty. Circulation. 2016;134(17):1247–56.
13. Borger MA, Murphy PM, Alam A, Fazel S, Maganti M, Armstrong S, et al. Initial results of the chordal-cutting operation for ischemic mitral regurgitation. J Thorac Cardiovasc Surg. 2007;133(6):1483–92.
14. Kron IL, Green GR, Cope JT. Surgical relocation of the posterior papillary muscle in chronic ischemic mitral regurgitation. Ann Thorac Surg. 2002;74(2):600–1.
15. Langer F, Rodriguez F, Ortiz S, Cheng A, Nguyen TC, Zasio MK, et al. Subvalvular repair: the key to repairing ischemic mitral regurgitation? Circulation. 2005;112(Suppl 9):I-383–9.
16. Langer F, Kunihara T, Hell K, Schramm R, Schmidt KI, Aicher D, et al. RING+STRING Successful repair technique for ischemic mitral regurgitation with severe leaflet tethering. Circulation. 2009;120(Suppl 1):S85–S91.
17. Nappi F, Lusini M, Spadaccio C, Nenna A, Covino E, Acar C, et al. Papillary muscle approximation versus restrictive annuloplasty alone for severe ischemic mitral regurgitation. J Am Coll Cardiol. 2016;67(20):2334–46.
18. Michler RE, Smith PK, Parides MK, Ailawadi G, Thourani V, Moskowitz AJ, et al. Two-year outcomes of surgical treatment of moderate ischemic mitral regurgitation. N Engl J Med. 2016;374(20):1932–41.
19. Nishimura RA, Otto CM, Bonow RO, Carabello BA, Erwin JP, Guyton RA, et al. AHA/ACC guideline for the management of patients with valvular heart disease: executive summary: a report of the American College of Cardiology/American Heart Association Task force on practice guidelines. Circulation. 2014;129:2440–92.
20. Nishimura RA, Otto CM, Bonow RO, Carabello BA, Erwin JP, Fleisher LA, et al. 2017 AHA/ACC focused update of the 2014 AHA/ACC guideline for the management of patients with valvular heart disease: a report of the American College of Cardiology/American Heart Association task force on clinical practice guidelines. Circulation. 2017;135(25):1159–95.
21. Goldstein D, Moskowitz AJ, Gelijns AC, Ailawadi G, Parides MK, Perrault LP, et al. Two-year outcomes of surgical treatment of severe ischemic mitral regurgitation. N Engl J Med. 2016;374(4):344–53.
22. Smith PK, Puskas JD, Ascheim DD, Voisine P, Gelijns AC, Moskowitz AJ, et al. Surgical treatment of moderate ischemic mitral regurgitation. N Engl J Med. 2014;371(23):2178–88.
23. Cooley DA, Collins HA, Morris GC Jr, Chapman DW. Ventricular aneurysm after myocardial infarction: surgical excision with use of temporary cardiopulmonary bypass. JAMA. 1958;167(5):557–60.
24. Cooley DA, Henly WS, Amad KH, Chapman DW. Ventricular aneurysm following myocardial infarction: results of surgical treatment. Ann Surg. 1959;150:595–612.

25. Favaloro RG, Effler DB, Groves LK, Westcott RN, Suarez E, Lozada J. Ventricular aneurysm--clinical experience. Ann Thorac Surg. 1968;63:227–45.
26. Dor V, Sabatier M, Di Donato M, Montiglio F, Toso A, Maioli M. Efficacy of endoventricular patch plasty in large postinfarction akinetic scar and severe left ventricular dysfunction: comparison with a series of large dyskinetic scars. J Thorac Cardiovasc Surg. 1998;116(1):50–9.
27. Dor V, Saab M, Coste P, Sabatier M, Montiglio F. Endoventricular patch plasties with septal exclusion for repair of ischemic left ventricle: technique, results and indications from a series of 781 cases. Jpn J Thorac Cardiovasc Surg. 1998;46(5):389–98.
28. Athanasuleas CL, Stanley AWH, Buckberg GD, Dor V, Di Donato M, Siler W. Surgical anterior ventricular endocardial restoration (SAVER) for dilated ischemic cardiomyopathy. Semin Thorac Cardiovasc Surg. 2001;13(4):448–58.
29. Yamaguchi A, Ino T, Adachi H, Mizuhara A, Murata S, Kamio H. Left ventricular end-systolic volume index in patients with ischemic cardiomyopathy predicts postoperative ventricular function. Ann Thorac Surg. 1995;60(4):1059–62.
30. Di Donato M, Toso A, Maioli M, Sabatier M, Stanley AWH, Dor V. Intermediate survival and predictors of death after surgical ventricular restoration. Semin Thorac Cardiovasc Surg. 2001;13(4):468–75.
31. Maxey TS, Reece TB, Ellman PI, Butler PD, Kern JA, Tribble CG, et al. Coronary artery bypass with ventricular restoration is superior to coronary artery bypass alone in patients with ischemic cardiomyopathy. J Thorac Cardiovasc Surg. 2004;127(2):428–34.
32. Menicanti L, Di Donato M. The Dor procedure: what has changed after fifteen years of clinical practice? J Thorac Cardiovasc Surg. 2002;124(5):886–90.
33. Isomura T, Horii T, Suma H, Buckberg GD. Septal anterior ventricular exclusion operation (Pacopexy) for ischemic dilated cardiomyopathy: treat form not disease. Eur J Cardio-Thorac Surg. 2006;29(Suppl 1):245–50.
34. Ueno T, Sakata R, Iguro Y, Yamamoto H, Ueno M, Ueno T, et al. Mid-term changes of left ventricular geometry and function after Dor, SAVE, and overlapping procedures. Eur J Cardio-Thorac Surg. 2007;32(1):52–7.
35. Jones RH, Velazquez EJ, Michler RE, Sopko G, Oh JK, O'Connor CM, et al. Coronary bypass surgery with or without surgical ventricular reconstruction. N Engl J Med. 2009;360(17):1705–17.

Chapter 10
LVAD Therapy

Teruhiko Imamura

Abstract Thus far, survival rate in patients with advanced heart failure has improved drastically due to the increased use of ventricular assist devices (LVADs). The most recent LVADs are implantable continuous-flow pumps, in contrast to older-generation extracorporeal pulsatile-flow devices. In Japan, LVAD implantation is indicated only as a bridge-to-transplantation, but is also allowed as therapy for non-transplant candidates in both Europe and the United States. Despite significant improvement in survival, there are still several unique LVAD-specific complications, which need further addressing: gastrointestinal bleeding, aortic insufficiency, pump thrombosis, and device-related infection.

Keywords Hemodynamics · Right heart failure · Unloading

10.1 Introduction

Despite advancements in heart failure-specific therapies, both short- and long-term survival in patients with advanced heart failure remains low [1]. The introduction of durable mechanical circulatory support in the form of left ventricular assist devices (LVADs) as an option for advanced heart failure patients has dramatically improved survival and quality of life for this vulnerable patient population [2]. Owing to an improvement in the technology of LVADs, including the latest HeartMate 3 pump, survival rates are improving to a level comparable to that of heart transplantation.

Nevertheless, there are several unique device-specific complications following implantation that remain problematic. In this review, I will describe the currently available devices, indications of LVAD therapy, hemodynamic effect of LVADs, and device-related adverse events.

T. Imamura (✉)
The Second Department of Internal Medicine, University of Toyama, Toyama, Japan

K. Kinugawa, T. Imamura (eds.), *Update of Non-Pharmacological Therapy for Heart Failure*, https://doi.org/10.1007/978-981-15-4843-7_10

10.2 Types of LVAD

Several iterations of LVADs have been introduced and innovated over the past two decades (Fig. 10.1) [3]. Older devices including extracorporeal and pulsatile devices such as NIPRO LVAD are still used in Japan for cases of cardiogenic shock as bridge-to-decision therapeutic option [4]. Figure 10.2 shows extracorporeal LVAD (Fig. 10.2a) and biventricular VAD (i.e., right heart support device and left heart support device; Fig. 10.2b). More recently, devices with continuous-flow technology are almost exclusively utilized as the pumps of choice in contemporary clinical settings. These types are further divided into axial-flow (HeartMate II [Abbott, Abbott Park, IL]) and centrifugal pumps (HeartMate 3 [Abbott, Abbott Park, IL]). Each device has a unique profile, and are often matched to patients based on optimal device–patient clinical compatibility.

Currently, EVAHEART2 (Sun Medical, Nagano, Japan), Jarvik 2000 (Jarvik Heart, Inc., New York, NY), HeartMate II, HVAD and HeartMate 3 are commercially available in Japan. In the United Stated, the only devices that are approved for commercial use are the HeartMate II, HeartMate 3, and HVAD (Medtronic, Minneapolis, Minnesota).

Of note, the Multicenter Study of MagLev Technology in Patients Undergoing Mechanical Circulatory Support Therapy With HeartMate 3 (MOMENTUM 3) has recently demonstrated that HeartMate 3, a fully magnetically levitated centrifugal-flow LVAD, has both higher survival and lower device-related adverse-event rates compared to the HeartMate II LVAD [5].

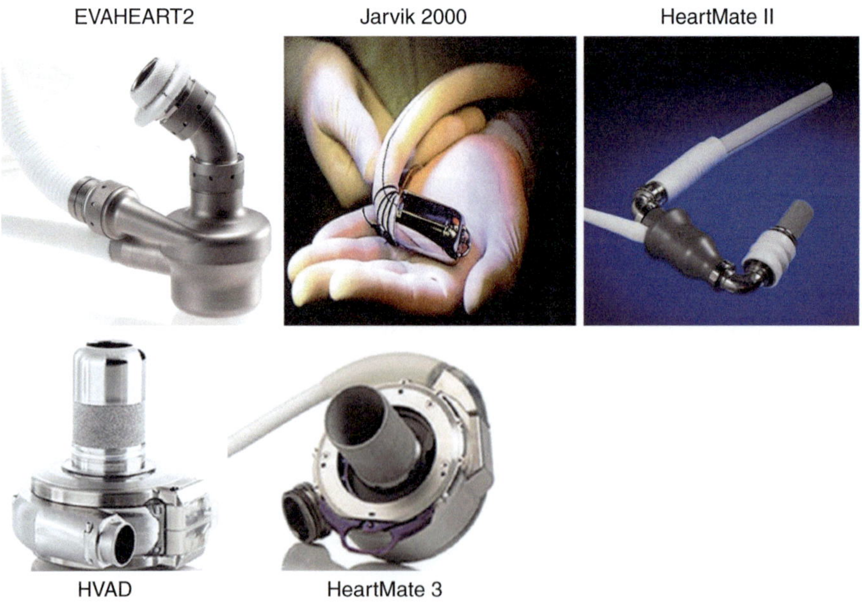

Fig. 10.1 Currently available left ventricular assist devices. Reused with alteration from reference [3] with permission

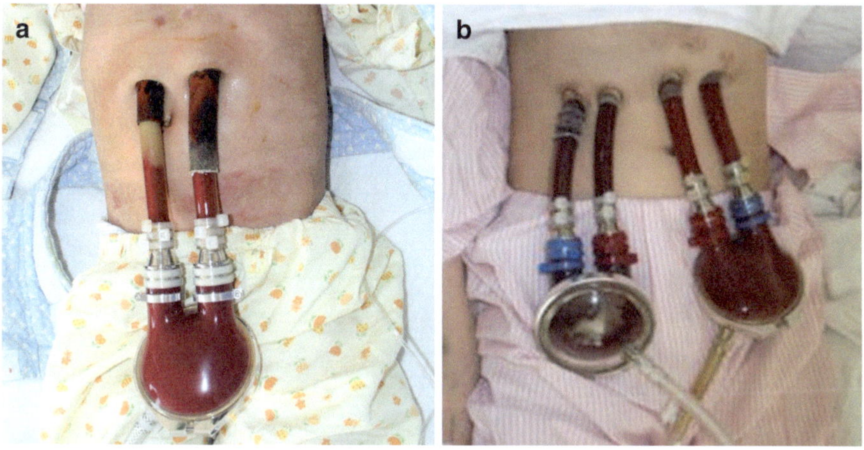

Fig. 10.2 Extracorporeal left ventricular assist device (**a**) and extracorporeal biventricular assist device (**b**)

10.3 Indications for LVAD Therapy

In Japan, the only indication for LVAD implantation is a bridge-to-heart transplantation [4]. In principle, patients should be listed for heart transplantation before LVAD implantation, and often will wait for several years with an LVAD prior to receiving a heart transplant. In both Europe and the United States, patients can undergo LVAD implantation as a definitive therapeutic option, when deemed not to be a candidate for heart transplantation (destination therapy) [2]. This indication is anticipated to receive approval in Japan in the near future. Some patients may experience reverse cardiac remodeling in the setting of both mechanical unloading and neurohormonal medical therapy, leading to significant myocardial recovery and an opportunity to proceed with device explantation (bridge-to-recovery) [6]. Models to predict myocardial recovery and the respective interventions which may increase the odds of recovery are active areas of investigation [7].

Other indication is bridge-to-decision. When patients' hemodynamics deteriorate immediately and we do not have sufficient time to discuss the eligibility of heart transplantation listing, extracorporeal LVAD might be indicated. Right heart support is required when biventricular heart failure is highly suspected particularly at the situation of fulminant myocarditis. Of note, we should be careful to implant extracorporeal LVAD in patients who would definitely not be candidates of heart transplant, given we in Japan are not allowed to implant LVAD as destination therapy indication thus far. If patients are listed for heart transplantation following extracorporeal LVAD implantation with improved end-organ function, we should consider the conversion to durable LVAD hopefully within several months to avoid complications such as infection at the cannulation sites, whose risk increases by months. The eligibility of device explantation due to cardiac reverse remodeling also should be considered within several months following extracorporeal LVAD implantation, by investigating the cardiac reserve.

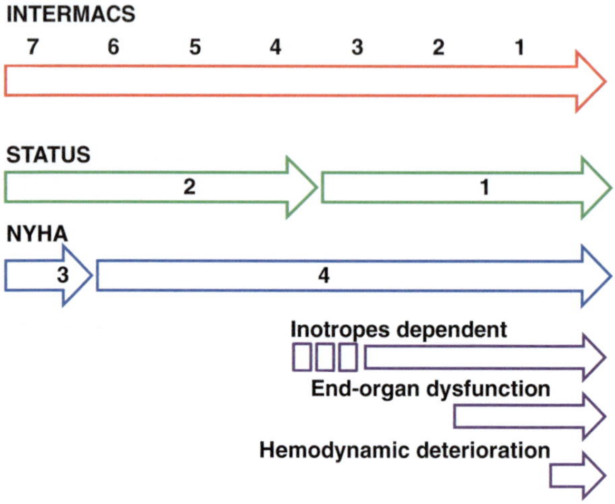

Fig. 10.3 Heart failure progression and grading. INTERMACS, interagency registry for mechanically assisted circulatory support; *NYHA* New York Heart Association. Advanced heart failure patients are stratified into seven INTERMACS profiles by clinical severity. Patients dependent on continuous intravenous inotropes are listed as status 1 for heart transplantation and have the advantage to receive a heart transplant before those with status 2, who are not inotrope-dependent

Optimal patient selection and timing of LVAD implantation may sometimes be challenging. As shown in Fig. 10.3, the INTERMACS profile provides seven grades to stratify the clinical acuity of the advanced heart failure patient [8]. When patients present with overt cardiogenic (INTERMACS 1 or 2), LVAD implantation becomes more risky with increased odds of perioperative complications and worse postoperative survival [9, 10]. On the contrary, meticulous consideration must be made to not implant these devices too early when patients are tolerating medical therapies with reasonable functional capacity, despite having severe structural heart disease [11]. In Japan, patients dependent on intravenous inotropes are listed for heart transplantation as status 1 and have the advantage to receive donor hearts compared to less sick (inotrope-free) patients assigned to status 2. Thus far, optimal timing for LVAD implantation should be considered at profile 3, when a patient has stable hemodynamics on intravenous inotropes. Improvement in device technology and perioperative management may eventually shift the optimal timing of LVAD into less sick populations (i.e., profile 4–6) in the near future [12].

10.4 Hemodynamic Changes Following LVAD Implantation

Given the mechanical unloading of the left ventricle (LV) and systemic circulatory support after LVAD implantation, we expect to see a decrease in pulmonary capillary wedge pressure along with an increase of cardiac output, providing more optimal hemodynamic profile to support end-organ circulation and improve functional capacity [3]. Due to the nature of continuous flow, arterial pulse pressure decreases.

Significant cardiac unloading usually results in a reduction of pulmonary artery pressures by reducing the afterload experienced by the pulmonary vasculature. Nevertheless, several patients following LVAD implantation may have inappropriately elevated diastolic pulmonary artery pressure despite reduced pulmonary artery wedge pressure, indicating fixed pulmonary vasculature damage [13, 14].

On the contrary to the left heart, right heart function seems to worsen longitudinally following LVAD implantation [15]. Despite a reduction in the afterload on right heart (i.e., pulmonary artery pressure), central venous pressures may remain unchanged due to increased venous return in the setting of restored cardiac output [16]. Increased LV unloading by incremental LVAD speed increases may eventually overwhelm the right ventricle, leading to leftward bowing of the intraventricular septum and eventual underfilling of the LV. Overall, postoperative right ventricular dysfunction can be more simply defined hemodynamically as an inappropriately elevated central venous pressure in the setting of normal pulmonary artery wedge pressure, often accompanied by signs of right-sided clinical congestion.

Interestingly, many LVAD patients in the setting of apparent clinical stability have non-optimized hemodynamics [16]. This has been found to be associated with worse clinical outcomes including an increased rate of heart failure readmissions and other hemocompatibility-related adverse events [17, 18]. Performing hemodynamic and echocardiographic ramp tests to optimize device speeds along with careful adjustment of guideline-directed medical therapy are important clinical strategies to improve outcomes in patients with LVADs (Fig. 10.4) [19]. Noninvasive methodologies to estimate hemodynamics including remote dielectric system and device-flow wave assessment might be useful tools to serially follow hemodynamics and guide device speed adjustments [20, 21]. This reduces the procedural risk to the patient by allowing for less right heart catheterizations in the setting of systemic anticoagulation.

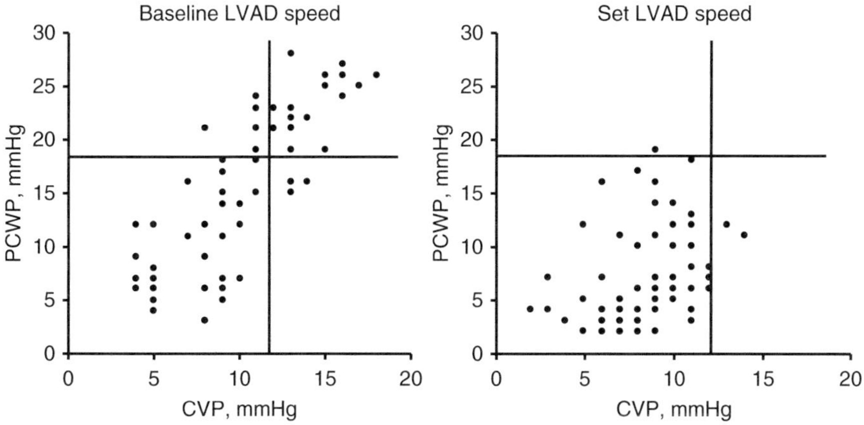

Fig. 10.4 Relationship between CVP and PCWP at baseline LVAD speed, and at set LVAD speed during hemodynamic ramp test. *CVP* central venous pressure, *PCWP* pulmonary capillary wedge pressure, *LVAD* left ventricular assist device. Many dots shift toward the left-lower direction (i.e., lower CVP and PCWP) when LVAD speed is adjusted following the hemodynamic ramp test

10.5 Unique Adverse Events During LVAD Support

10.5.1 Aortic Insufficiency

Eccentric regurgitant flow through the aortic valve often occurs not only at diastole but also at systolic during LVAD support. The exact mechanism of de novo aortic insufficiency (AI) remains unclear. It is postulated that aortic root degeneration due to reduced arterial pulsatility and prolonged aortic valve closure during continuous left ventricular unloading may contribute to the development and progression of AI [22–24]. Following the development of AI, both pulmonary capillary wedge pressure and central venous pressure increase. Incremental LVAD speed increases may worsen the severity of AI over time by increasing regurgitant flow, although temporary speed increases may improve hemodynamics and help relieve clinical congestion in the short term [25].

Patients with AI have worse long-term survival, higher readmission rates, and lower exercise capacity compared to those without AI [23, 26]. Our team recently proposed a novel methodology to quantify the severity of AI by using Doppler echocardiography obtained at the LVAD outflow graft [27]. We found that conventional visual estimation seems to underestimate the severity of AI, possibly delaying potential therapeutic interventions [28].

For the management of mild AI, it is recommended keep the LVAD speed lower to allow for aortic valve opening [29]. Recently, transcatheter aortic valve replacement (TAVR) has been used as a nonsurgical technique to treat severe AI [30]. Long-term outcomes of TAVR for the treatment of severe AI are unclear, but exists as a promising therapy to potentially improve symptoms and survival in patients who otherwise would be poor surgical re-operative candidates.

10.5.2 Gastrointestinal Bleeding

Gastrointestinal bleeding (GIB) is one of the major causes of readmissions during LVAD support in both Europe and the United States. The specific etiology and pathophysiology of GIB in LVAD patients remain largely unknown. The rate of GIB post-LVAD implant, however, is surprisingly low in Japanese patients [4]. One of the accepted mechanisms of GIB post-LVAD is the development of arteriovenous malformations located on the surface of gastrointestinal tract. In addition to systemic anticoagulation and antiplatelet therapies [31], acquired von Willebrand disease and the development of arteriovenous malformation due to activated inflammatory and angiogenesis systems may be the predominant causes of GIB in LVAD patients [32].

When GIB occurs, discontinuation of antiplatelet and anticoagulation agents are often the mainstays of therapy, in addition to endoscopic interventions performed to identify and treat active bleeding areas from arteriovenous malformations. Although there are no definitive therapies to prevent GIB in LVAD patients, omega-3 fatty acid and digoxin administration have been recently proposed as potential primary prevention therapies [33], albeit the data available is only observational at this time. For secondary prevention, octreotide, thalidomide, and androgen are therapies often used for refractory bleeding episodes [34].

10.5.3 Pump Thrombosis

Pump thrombosis is one of the most critical complications which may occur during LVAD support, and often results in systemic thromboembolism as well as device malfunction. This complication unfortunately can result in both fatal disability and critical hemodynamic deterioration [35].

Early and accurate diagnosis of pump thrombosis is sometimes challenging. Patients with pump thrombosis suffer from atypical heart failure symptoms and often have abnormally elevated serum lactate dehydrogenase levels. Furthermore, device log files may suggest dramatic increases in power along with low flows. Echocardiographic ramp studies may be considered for those with suspected pump thrombosis in patients with HeartMate II LVADs [36]. In the event of device thrombosis, the ramp study would show an inability to decompress the LV cavity along with sustained aortic valve opening despite increasing the device speed. This technique, however, is less accurate in diagnosing thrombosis in HVAD devices.

When pump thrombosis is suspected, intensified anticoagulation therapy with intravenous heparinization should be initiated. Pump exchange or urgent heart transplantation have historically been the preferred management strategies employed for device thrombosis. Given data showing improved clinical outcomes following device exchange owing to the recently developed minimally invasive surgical technique using subcostal approach, device exchanges can be performed with considerably less risk compared to prior methods which required re-do sternotomy [37]. Of note, the most recently developed device, HeartMate 3 LVAD, showed an extremely low pump thrombosis rate [5], providing a much-needed advancement in the era of durable mechanical circulatory support.

Acknowledgment

Conflicts of Interest None

References

1. Rose EA, Gelijns AC, Moskowitz AJ, et al. Long-term use of a left ventricular assist device for end-stage heart failure. N Engl J Med. 2001;345(20):1435–43.
2. Kormos RL, Cowger J, Pagani FD, et al. The society of thoracic surgeons intermacs database annual report: evolving indications, outcomes, and scientific partnerships. J Heart Lung Transplant. 2019;38(2):114–26.
3. Imamura T, Chung B, Nguyen A, Sayer G, Uriel N. Clinical implications of hemodynamic assessment during left ventricular assist device therapy. J Cardiol. 2018;71(4):352–8.

4. Nakatani T, Sase K, Oshiyama H, et al. Japanese registry for mechanically assisted circulatory support: first report. J Heart Lung Transplant. 2017;36(10):1087–96.
5. Mehra MR, Uriel N, Naka Y, et al. A fully magnetically levitated left ventricular assist device – final report. N Engl J Med. 2019;380(17):1618–27.
6. Imamura T, Kinugawa K, Hatano M, et al. Preoperative beta-blocker treatment is a key for deciding left ventricular assist device implantation strategy as a bridge to recovery. J Artif Organs. 2014;17(1):23–32.
7. Imamura T, Kinugawa K, Nitta D, et al. Novel scoring system using postoperative cardiopulmonary exercise testing predicts future explantation of left ventricular assist device. Circ J. 2015;79(3):560–6.
8. Kinugawa K. How to treat stage D heart failure? – when to implant left ventricular assist devices in the era of continuous flow pumps? Circ J. 2011;75(9):2038–45.
9. Kirklin JK, Pagani FD, Kormos RL, et al. Eighth annual INTERMACS report: special focus on framing the impact of adverse events. J Heart Lung Transplant. 2017;36(10):1080–6.
10. Imamura T, Kinugawa K, Shiga T, et al. Novel risk scoring system with preoperative objective parameters gives a good prediction of 1-year mortality in patients with a left ventricular assist device. Circ J. 2012;76(8):1895–903.
11. Starling RC, Estep JD, Horstmanshof DA, et al. Risk assessment and comparative effectiveness of left ventricular assist device and medical management in ambulatory heart failure patients: the ROADMAP study 2-year results. JACC Heart Fail. 2017;5(7):518–27.
12. Imamura T, Kinugawa K, Nitta D, Kinoshita O, Nawata K, Ono M. Is cardiopulmonary exercise testing essential to indicate ventricular assist device implantation in patients with INTERMACS profile 4-7? J Artif Organs. 2016;19(3):226–32.
13. Imamura T, Kim G, Raikhelkar J, et al. Decoupling between diastolic pulmonary arterial pressure and pulmonary arterial wedge pressure at incremental left ventricular assist device (LVAD) speeds is associated with worse prognosis after LVAD implantation. J Card Fail. 2018;24(9):575–82.
14. Imamura T, Chung B, Nguyen A, et al. Decoupling between diastolic pulmonary artery pressure and pulmonary capillary wedge pressure as a prognostic factor after continuous flow ventricular assist device implantation. Circ Heart Fail. 2017;10(9):e003882.
15. Imamura T, Kinugawa K, Kato N, et al. Late-onset right ventricular failure in patients with preoperative small left ventricle after implantation of continuous flow left ventricular assist device. Circ J. 2014;78(3):625–33.
16. Uriel N, Sayer G, Addetia K, et al. Hemodynamic ramp tests in patients with left ventricular assist devices. JACC Heart Fail. 2016;4(3):208–17.
17. Imamura T, Nguyen A, Kim G, et al. Optimal haemodynamics during left ventricular assist device support are associated with reduced haemocompatibility-related adverse events. Eur J Heart Fail. 2019;21(5):655–62.
18. Imamura T, Jeevanandam V, Kim G, et al. Optimal hemodynamics during left ventricular assist device support are associated with reduced readmission rates. Circ Heart Fail. 2019;12(2):e005094.
19. Uriel N, Burkhoff D, Rich JD, et al. Impact of hemodynamic ramp test-guided HVAD speed and medication adjustments on clinical outcomes. Circ Heart Fail. 2019;12(4):e006067.
20. Uriel N, Sayer G, Imamura T, et al. Relationship between noninvasive assessment of lung fluid volume and invasively measured cardiac hemodynamics. J Am Heart Assoc. 2018;7(22):e009175.
21. Grinstein J, Rodgers D, Kalantari S, et al. HVAD waveform analysis as a noninvasive marker of pulmonary capillary wedge pressure: a first step toward the development of a smart left ventricular assist device pump. ASAIO J. 2018;64(1):10–5.
22. Letsou GV, Connelly JH, Delgado RM 3rd, et al. Is native aortic valve commissural fusion in patients with long-term left ventricular assist devices associated with clinically important aortic insufficiency? J Heart Lung Transplant. 2006;25(4):395–9.
23. Imamura T, Kinugawa K, Fujino T, et al. Aortic insufficiency in patients with sustained left ventricular systolic dysfunction after axial flow assist device implantation. Circ J. 2015;79(1):104–11.

24. Imamura T, Kinugawa K, Nitta D, et al. Advantage of pulsatility in left ventricular reverse remodeling and aortic insufficiency prevention during left ventricular assist device treatment. Circ J. 2015;79(9):1994–9.
25. Sayer G, Sarswat N, Kim GH, et al. The hemodynamic effects of aortic insufficiency in patients supported with continuous-flow left ventricular assist devices. J Card Fail. 2017;23(7):545–51.
26. Cowger J, Pagani FD, Haft JW, Romano MA, Aaronson KD, Kolias TJ. The development of aortic insufficiency in left ventricular assist device-supported patients. Circ Heart Fail. 2010;3(6):668–74.
27. Grinstein J, Kruse E, Sayer G, et al. Accurate quantification methods for aortic insufficiency severity in patients with LVAD: role of diastolic flow acceleration and systolic-to-diastolic peak velocity ratio of outflow cannula. JACC Cardiovasc Imaging. 2016;9(6):641–51.
28. Grinstein J, Kruse E, Sayer G, et al. Novel echocardiographic parameters of aortic insufficiency in continuous-flow left ventricular assist devices and clinical outcome. J Heart Lung Transplant. 2016;35(8):976–85.
29. Imamura T, Kinugawa K, Nitta D, Hatano M, Ono M. Opening of aortic valve during exercise is key to preventing development of aortic insufficiency during ventricular assist device treatment. ASAIO J. 2015;61(5):514–9.
30. Yehya A, Rajagopal V, Meduri C, et al. Short-term results with transcatheter aortic valve replacement for treatment of left ventricular assist device patients with symptomatic aortic insufficiency. J Heart Lung Transplant. 2019;38:920–6.
31. Tabit CE, Chen P, Kim GH, et al. Elevated angiopoietin-2 level in patients with continuous-flow left ventricular assist devices leads to altered angiogenesis and is associated with higher nonsurgical bleeding. Circulation. 2016;134(2):141–52.
32. Imamura T, Kinugawa K, Uriel N. Therapeutic strategy for gastrointestinal bleeding in patients with left ventricular assist device. Circ J. 2018;82(12):2931–8.
33. Imamura T, Nguyen A, Rodgers D, et al. Omega-3 therapy is associated with reduced gastrointestinal bleeding in patients with continuous-flow left ventricular assist device. Circ Heart Fail. 2018;11(10):e005082.
34. Juricek C, Imamura T, Nguyen A, et al. Long-acting octreotide reduces the recurrence of gastrointestinal bleeding in patients with a continuous-flow left ventricular assist device. J Card Fail. 2018;24(4):249–54.
35. Nguyen AB, Uriel N, Adatya S. New challenges in the treatment of patients with left ventricular support: LVAD thrombosis. Curr Heart Fail Rep. 2016;13(6):302–9.
36. Uriel N, Morrison KA, Garan AR, et al. Development of a novel echocardiography ramp test for speed optimization and diagnosis of device thrombosis in continuous-flow left ventricular assist devices: the Columbia ramp study. J Am Coll Cardiol. 2012;60(18):1764–75.
37. Kitahara H, Raikhelkar J, Kim G, et al. A subcostal approach is favorable compared to sternotomy for left ventricular assist device exchange field of research: artificial heart (clinical). J Artif Organs. 2019;11

Chapter 11
Heart Transplantation

Minoru Ono

Abstract Although many non-pharmacological therapies have been introduced into the treatment of advanced heart failure, heart transplantation is still a gold standard for end-stage heart failure with a considerably high quality of life and relatively long survival period. In this chapter, I will describe the indication, management, and complications of heart transplantation.

Keywords Calcineurin inhibitors · Rejection · Mycophenolate mofetil · Coronary artery vasculopathy

11.1 Introduction

Since the first heart transplantation in 1967, more than 130,000 patients underwent heart transplantation [1]. Introduction of cyclosporine to heart transplantation dramatically improved the prognosis in the early 1980s. Establishment of safe and reliable triple immunosuppressive regimen accelerated worldwide spread of this treatment. Standardized cardiac biopsy grading as results of collaborative work in International Society for Heart Transplantation in 1990 [2] enabled uniform diagnosis of the grade of cellular rejection. Two epoch-making progresses in immunosuppressive drug were encountered in the 1990s, Tacrolimus and mycophenolate mofetil, which further improved long-term results after heart transplantation. Around the starting year of millennium, sirolimus and everolimus were introduced to heart transplantation. Coronary artery vasculopathy (CAV), which hitherto was progressive end-stage injury of coronary artery, was found to be treatable thanks to the inhibitory function of proliferation signal of these drugs. Antibody-mediated rejection (AMR), also referred to as humoral rejection, was hard to diagnose precisely and treat effectively. Recently, detection of anti-HLA antibody became possible. Heart transplantation in early days utilized the heart from non-heart beating

M. Ono (✉)
Department of Cardiovascular Surgery, University of Tokyo, Tokyo, Japan
e-mail: mono-tky@umin.ac.jp

K. Kinugawa, T. Imamura (eds.), *Update of Non-Pharmacological Therapy for Heart Failure*, https://doi.org/10.1007/978-981-15-4843-7_11

donor. A recent great effort to tackle with severe brain-dead donor shortage led to utilization of the heart from non-heart beating donor again [3].

11.2 Indications

Generally accepted indications for heart transplantation were listed in Table 11.1 [4]. End-stage heart disease is encountered in various types of diseases encompassing so-called cardiomyopathy including both ischemic and idiopathic etiologies. Idiopathic dilated cardiomyopathy is the most popular in Western countries, but hypertrophic (particularly, dilated-phase), restrictive, and postpartum cardiomyopathies are also included. Secondary cardiomyopathy, such as drug-induced, post-myocarditis, autoimmune-related, may be indicated for heart transplantation. End-stage heart failure is also encountered in congenital and valvular heart disease. Retransplantation is indicated in limited number of patients due to insufficient organ donation.

End-stage condition is defined by impaired heart function and poor exercise tolerance. Generally accepted level of condition by which transplantation is considered is history of New York Heart Association functional class IV symptoms which are resistant to optimal medical or surgical treatment and accompanied by repeated episodes of hospital admission due to heart failure. Cardiopulmonary exercise testing is a reliable modality to confirm the level of depression of daily activity. Maximal $VO_2 < 10–14$ mL/kg/min is generally accepted level of exercise impairment [5, 6]. Recurrent episodes of ventricular arrhythmia which is refractory to all available therapeutic modalities is also indicated.

There is no generally accepted consensus on the upper age limit for heart transplantation. The upper age limit is 65 years in many countries, but this upper limit is not an absolute, but rather relies on the treatment team's discretion. The upper age is balanced between the numbers of organ donations and waiting patients, and chronological age may not be so good an indicator for recovery of social activity as physical one. Recently, 2.0% of adult heart transplantation were performed in patients with age over 70 years in the 2019 ISHLT registry report [1].

Table 11.1 Generally accepted indications for cardiac transplantation [4]

1. End-stage heart disease not amenable to other medical or surgical therapy that limits 1-year survival less than 50%
2. NYHA class III to IV symptoms on optimal medical therapy
3. Age is generally 65 years or younger
4. Healthy apart from heart disease
5. Emotionally stable, well-motivated to resume active lifestyle
6. Compliant with medical advice
7. Supportive family/companions willing and able to make similar long-term commitments

Adherence to physician's advice and medications is an important factor which makes post-transplant life more active and less problematic. Assessment of personal qualities is not always easy, but should be conducted thoroughly prior to consideration to transplant listing. Strong and supportive family environment is an important factor which enables a patient to tolerate and overcome post-transplant stresses and issues.

There are several medical conditions which may lead to no benefit or even to unsatisfactory outcomes. There are some absolute contraindications to heart transplantation. Basically, advanced dysfunction of multiple organs (cerebral, pulmonary, renal, and hepatic), untreatable active infection, malignant disease with a limited life expectancy, psychiatric illnesses which are likely to interfere with compliance, and other medical conditions which negatively impact and complicate post-transplant life (insulin-dependent diabetes mellitus, advanced peripheral vascular disease, and other systemic illnesses). A patient with severe other organ damage may be a candidate for multiple organ transplantation, such as heart–lung, heart–kidney, and heart–liver transplantation.

11.3 Patient Management

The treatment and management of a patient awaiting heart transplantation is a starting point of patient care. Waiting time for heart transplantation has been lengthened worldwide. Considering end-stage condition of a transplantation candidate, careful patient management is mandatory to reduce wait-list death as low as we could. Multidisciplinary approach is mandatory to maintain patient hemodynamics and symptoms in a reasonable condition. Patient management strategies consist of education on dietary habit, luxury grocery item and lifestyle, pharmacological therapy, electrophysiological intervention, and mechanical circulatory support. Tobacco use should be prohibited, and alcohol intake should be avoided. Sodium and water intake are restricted to a predetermined level. Angiotensin-converting enzyme inhibitor and beta-blocker are mainstay for treatment of systolic dysfunction, which sometimes provides a patient with a chance of reverse remodeling. Diuretics is prescribed based on the level of water retention and congestion. Although loop diuretics and thiazide are commonly used, tolvaptan, which is vasopressin receptor-2 antagonist is reported to be safe and effective to remove circulating volume without disturbing electrolyte balance. Beta-blocker and amiodarone are administered to treat ventricular arrhythmias. Beta-blocker and digoxin are choice of medicine for treatment of tachycardia. Ivabradine, which is HCN4 channel blocker, is an emerging drug which can effectively control sinus tachycardia. Anticoagulation therapy by using warfarin is conducted to avoid cardiogenic thromboembolic episode.

Cardiac resynchronization therapy (CRT) is widely adopted for a patient with severely reduced left ventricular systolic function accompanied by ventricular dyssynchrony. Readjustment of resynchronization timing is necessary according to the progression of the native disease or other relevant conditions. Implantable cardioverter defibrillator (ICD) is routinely used in a patient with lethal ventricular arrhythmia. Heart transplantation candidate frequently experiences ventricular tachycardia and even ventricular fibrillation for which ICD is a lifesaving device. Many patients in a waiting list are implanted with combination of CRT and ICD (CRT-D).

Ventricular assist device (VAD) has been becoming popular due to its rapid technological advances. Until the mid-2000s paracorporeal VAD or implantable, but large-size pulsatile VAD were used for bridge to transplantation (BTT). Emergence of continuous-flow VAD (CFVAD) changed the clinical landscape completely due to its much smaller size and longer durability and reliability. The ratio of patients who underwent transplantation by BTT was 25–30% range in the United States until 2008. It increased abruptly up to 50% after approval of HeartMate II as BTT indication. BTT by implanting CFVAD is far more popular and essential in Japan due to severe donor shortage. Since the first CFVADs (EVAHERT and DuraHeart) were approved in 2011, BTT ratio has been much higher with more than 90% [7].

11.4 Matching of Recipient and Donor

Several factors are taken into account for matching of donor and recipient to achieve successful heart transplantation. Blood type should be identical or compatible, although blood type-incompatible heart transplantation is possible in an infant. Body size is also considered, and commonly acceptable donor body size mismatch is from −20% to +30% to a recipient. Body weight is the most popular indicator of body size for heart transplantation, but other factors may be utilized. Recently, predicted heart mass was reported to be the most reliable size matching parameter [8]. Prospective crossmatch is desirable to avoid hyperacute rejection. This is routinely adopted in Japan, which leads to significant reduction of in-hospital death. Prospective crossmatch may not be necessarily practical in other countries or regions. To reduce hyperacute rejection virtual crossmatch is an effective detection method of donor specific antibody (DSA) in a recipient [9].

11.5 Operative Techniques

There are two techniques to transplant the heart: orthotopic and heterotopic. In this chapter only orthotopic transplantation is described. General anesthesia is induced and pulmonary artery catheter may be or may not be inserted. It is recommended to insert pulmonary artery catheter in a patient with confirmed or possible pulmonary hypertension. Transesophageal echocardiography is an essential tool to monitor heart function and residual air bubbles in heart chambers. Recipient median sternotomy incision is started in keeping with donor preparation and cardiotomy. Transportation time from the donated hospital should be also taken into account.

Preparation of a recipient chest is usually ready within 30 min for primary chest. For a redo sternotomy case, an extra time to dissect and expose the heart is considered. In particular, preparation of a recipient chest takes much longer time when the patient is on a ventricular assist device.

Heart can be dissected and exposed without cardiopulmonary bypass (CPB) support, or CPB support can be initiated earlier to make dissection safer and faster. Timely preparation of recipient chest is mandatory to save time of donor heart as short as possible. Recipient heart is to be explanted soon after arrival of a donor heart to the operating room. Donor heart is examined as to patent foramen ovale (PFO) and incision on the left atrial appendage (LAA) which is usually made during flashing the donor lungs. PFO and LAA incision are suture-closed if necessary.

Technique and sequence of anastomoses are varying by surgeon's preference and experience. The classical technique is biatrial anastomosis, also referred to as Lower–Shumway method. Right atria are anastomosed to each other in the body of right atrium. This technique has several advantages such as enabling faster and easier anastomosis. But, this classical technique has been less frequently used due to higher incidence of significant tricuspid regurgitation and sick sinus syndrome requiring pacemaker implantation late after transplantation. Bicaval anastomosis, in which right atrial anastomosis is conducted at each vena cava level, has replaced the classical technique. Kitamura et al. reported efficacy of modified bicaval anastomosis in which the continuity of both cavae is preserved by remaining posterior wall right atrium [10]. This technique is superior to the original bicaval technique particularly in a case with a big size discrepancy of inferior vena cava.

The most important factor for transplantation surgery is to keep ischemic time of donor heart less than 4 h. Sufficient reperfusion is continued to confirm sufficient recovery of transplanted heart. Infusion of inotropes and phosphodiesterase 3 inhibitor is initiated well before weaning from CPB. Atrial pacing is used if necessary. Nitric oxide (NO) inhalation should be always ready for use, and inhalation is started routinely or if necessary according to surgeon or anesthesiologist policy or decision. Vasoplegia is frequently encountered at the time of weaning from CPB particularly in a patient who was on ventricular assist device for a long period. Norepinephrine and/or vasopressin is titrated to raise blood pressure, and methylene blue may be indicated in an extreme case.

11.6 Postoperative Management in Acute Phase

A transplanted patient is transferred to a room designated for care of transplantation patient in the ICU. Postoperative care and hemodynamic monitoring are the same as regular open-heart surgery. Strict isolation is no longer necessary, although thorough hand-washing and wearing a mask are required. EKG, echocardiography, and X-ray machines are thoroughly cleaned before entering the room.

Sinus tachycardia is usually seen after heart transplantation resulting from sympathetic denervation with heart rate over 100 beats per minute. Tachycardia can be left untreated in an acute phase, but reduction of heart rate may be reasonable by beta-blockers once the hemodynamic condition is stabilized. Bradycardia less than 60 beats per minute may be encountered, in that case atrial pacing is considered by temporary epicardial pacing leads. Diastolic dysfunction is seen almost always to a varying degree, and it is frequently experienced in a patient whose ischemic time is long or in case that the size of the transplanted heart is small. In this scenario, high central venous pressure and low cardiac output with preserved left ventricular systolic function and small left ventricle are generally observed combination in a hemodynamic and echocardiographic examinations. This marginal hemodynamic condition is usually improved in about a month. NO inhalation is titrated down by monitoring pulmonary artery pressure and cardiac output, and can be usually stopped over a night. If a patient present with persistent pulmonary hypertension, pharmacological treatment for pulmonary hypertension is necessary. Phosphodiesterase 5 inhibitors (sildenafil and tadalafil) are choice of drug for this purpose because endothelin receptor antagonist (bosentan) is shown to have significant interaction with calcineurin inhibitors.

Mechanical circulatory support may be required in case of primary graft dysfunction (PGD). PGD is caused by multifactorial reasons which include prolonged ischemic time, inadequate preservation (temperature, preservation solution), inherent donor heart disease, small donor heart and so on. Graft dysfunction may be caused by secondary reasons such as hyperacute rejection, recipient pulmonary hypertension, and massive transfusion. Intraaortic balloon pump (IABP) is a device of the first choice for this purpose, and the majority of hemodynamic impairment is recovered. If the hemodynamic condition is not sufficiently supported by IABP, extracorporeal membrane oxygenation (ECMO) is considered, particularly for right ventricular failure. Extracorporeal VAD or Impella may be required in a more advanced systolic dysfunction.

11.7 Rejection

Acute cellular rejection is a major target for examination and treatment after heart transplantation. Noninvasive methods were reported, but the most reliable and definitive method to detect cellular rejection is endomyocardial biopsy. Standardized cardiac biopsy grading was proposed by Billingham in 1990 [2], which consisted of four grading (Table 11.2). This grading system was revised in 2004 [11] (Table 11.2). Immunosuppression is tailored and optimized according to the grade of rejection. When severe level of cellular rejection (grade 3A/grade 2R or higher) is observed, methylprednisolone pulse therapy is performed along with optimization or conversion of current immunosuppressive regimen. Incidence of cellular rejection is higher within 6 months after heart transplantation, so the majority of heart transplantation program perform frequent biopsies in early phase. Cellular rejection can occur late after transplantation. Tight adherence to immunosuppressive regimen, though in a

Table 11.2 Grading of acute cellular rejection after heart transplantation

Histologic grade	Extent of inflammatory infiltrate	Myocyte injury
Grade 0/0R	Absent or rare interstitial lymphocytes	Absent
Grade 1A/1R Focal mild	Focal perivascular interstitial infiltrate of activated lymphocytes; Infiltrates usually become smaller on subsequent levels	Absent
Grade 1B/1R Diffuse mild	Few activated lymphocytes between myocytes	Absent No eosinophils or muscle damage
Grade 2/1R Focal moderate	Single focus of activated lymphocytes, which may include eosinophils macrophages and few plasma cells	Focal myocyte damage
Grade 3A/2R	2 or more foci of infiltrate, each similar to Grade 2	Multifocal myocyte damage
Grade 3B and 4/3R	Rarely seen with current therapy; manifested by diffuse infiltrates with edema and hemorrhage in severe rejection	Multifocal myocyte damage

reduced dose, is mandatory for prevention of cellular rejection in late phase. Many programs omit regular endomyocardial biopsy late after (e.g., 10 years) transplantation due to rare occurrence of rejection.

Another mode of rejection is AMR. Hyperacute rejection is an extreme expression of AMR which is caused by high titer of preformed DSA. AMR, not hyperacute rejection, may occur early after transplantation, which may exhibit sustained low output syndrome or gradual decrease of transplanted heart function. High index of suspicion is of utmost importance in this situation. Emergent biopsy may be useful to detect positive complement deposit (C3d, C4d) or other characteristic histological findings of AMR. Detection of DSA may be also helpful. Prompt intervention is mandatory in the majority of cases, including either or combination of high-dose intravenous administration of immunoglobulin, plasma exchange, and rituximab. AMR may occur at any timing after transplantation. Recent recommendation is to monitor anti-HLA antibody, particularly DSA, regularly at the time of biopsy admission or clinic visit.

11.8 Immunosuppressive Treatment

Triple drug regimen is a standard immunosuppressive treatment for heart transplantation to prevent rejection. Calcineurin inhibitor (CNI) is a main immunosuppressant acting by blocking T cell expansion through inhibition of IL-2 production. There are two kinds of CNI: cyclosporine and tacrolimus. Tacrolimus is a preferred CNI in current practice in the majority of program due to more efficacy to inhibit cellular rejection. In combination with CNI antimetabolite is used. Azathioprine was used for this purpose. Mycophenolate mofetil (MMF) has replaced azathioprine almost completely due to its stronger immunosuppressive potency. MMF blocks inosine monophosphate dehydrogenase I/II, thereby inhibits lymphocyte proliferation through inhibition of de novo DNA synthesis. Steroid is a third drug which is used in many situations during the course of heart transplantation. One gram of methylprednisolone is administered intravenously just prior to reperfusion of the transplanted heart to block allogeneic response and reperfusion injury. Intravenous administration of methylprednisolone (usually 125 mg) every 8 h is adopted widely as initial immunosuppression early after transplantation before starting CNI and antimetabolite.

Mammalian target of rapamycin (mTOR) inhibitor (sirolimus and everolimus) is an emerging immunosuppressant. mTOR inhibitors act as an inhibition of proliferation of lymphocytes and smooth muscle cells. This drug has multipotent functions such as complementary or alternative drug to CNI to protect renal function or MMF in case of thrombocytopenia or gastrointestinal complications, protective to cytomegalovirus (CMV) infection, rescue therapy of intractable acute cellular rejection, and inhibition of progression of CAV [12]. mTOR inhibitor is usually administered several months or years after transplantation when indicated. De novo administration of mTOR inhibitor after heart transplantation is not generally accepted due to its side effect (wound healing impairment).

Induction immunosuppression is conducted in one-third to half of transplantation. Polyclonal antilymphocyte globulin or antithymocyte globulin had been used for this purpose, but they are less indicated now. IL-2 receptor antagonist (basiliximab) is the most frequently selected recently due to its less side effects.

11.9 Infection Control

Prophylactic anti-infection treatment is routinely conducted after heart transplantation, and consists of prophylaxis to viruses and fungi. Bacterial or fungal infection is seen early after heart transplantation as in regular open-heart surgery. Particularly, expansion of smoldering infection at driveline or pump site in a patient on ventricular assist device may occur even after removal of the device. Consultation to infection control team and choice of adequate sensitive antibiotics are mandatory in this situation. Additional debridement or omental flap coverage if necessary may be performed simultaneously at the time of transplantation surgery to prevent expansion of infection. General precaution is sufficient to prevent extrinsic infection. Unnecessarily long placement of catheter should be avoided.

CMV may be transmitted and activated in a seronegative recipient 2–6 weeks after transplantation. Because transfusion may lead to CMV infection, white blood cell depletion filter should be used and CMV negative blood may be preferably prepared for a seronegative patient. CMV immunoglobulin may be used to inhibit reactivation of CMV. Prophylactic administration of ganciclovir is considered particularly in case of high-risk combination (donor seropositive/recipient seronegative). Otherwise, there is no consensus on which is better, prophylactic administration or preemptive treatment. Regular monitoring of CMV antigenemia or DNA is mandatory during acute phase after transplantation. A recipient is asymptomatic during early stage of viremia. Hepatitis, pneumonia or enterocolitis may develop as CMV disease.

Epstein Barr virus (EBV) may cause serious complications after transplantation. EBV is transmitted from EBV seropositive donor or blood transfusion to a seronegative recipient. Proliferation of EBV causes various types of disease, such as infectious mononucleosis, chronic infection of bone marrow, malignant B cell lymphoma (posttransplant lymphoproliferative disease: PTLD), and hemophagocytic syndrome. Children and young adults are more susceptible to EBV infection and progression to the diseases because many of them are seronegative for EBV. Some patients can become free of infection just by reducing dose of immunosuppressant, but infection may progress to a higher level of disease (chronic infection and/or PTLD) in the other patients for whom chemotherapy is required (single rituximab or R-CHOP).

Fungal infection may develop several months after transplantation, including candidiasis, aspergillosis, pneumocystosis, and cryptococcosis. Candidiasis may occur on the skin, in the mouth, throat and esophagus, and in the eye. Aspergillosis occurs in the lung, and sometimes quite difficult to treat, particularly in case of invasive infection. Cryptococcosis may be seen in the lung, the brain and the whole body.

11.10 Other Complications

CAV is seen about 50% of recipients at 10 years after transplantation [1]. CAV is progressive disease and one of major causes of death seen several years and later after transplantation. This specific pathology is characterized by diffuse thickening of intima from large epicardial artery down to peripheral small vessels, and thought to be caused by chronically continuing rejection process. Diagnostic accuracy of CAV by conventional coronary angiography [13] is low, and intravascular ultrasound (IVUS) [14] or optical coherence tomography [15] is more sensitive and accurate to grade the severity of the disease. There are two popular grading criteria for CAV, International Society for Heart and Lung Transplantation (ISHLT) classification based on coronary angiography [13] and Stanford classification based on IVUS evaluation [14]. Other noninvasive method measuring coronary flow reserve by echocardiography [16] or computed tomography were reported. Because other comorbidities, such as hypertension, hyperlipidemia, and diabetes mellitus, may accelerate CAV disease process, adequate pharmacological treatment on these comorbidities is essential to avoid or slow down the disease progression. Statin and aspirin have been used empirically with hope of reducing the risk of coronary events. Reportedly, mTOR inhibitors may stop, or even reverse CAV disease process [17]. This prompted addition or conversion to mTOR inhibitors when CAV is identified, or even for prophylaxis of CAV. Coronary artery bypass surgery or percutaneous coronary intervention are considered in a selected case with localized stenosis.

Malignancy is a leading cause of death 5 years and later after transplantation, accounting for 20% and prevalence is increased as the time elapses [1]. According to the most recent registry report from ISHLT [1], 27.7% of patients suffered from some type of malignancy in 10 year survivors. Skin malignancy is the most frequent one, followed by solid organ malignancy in 10.2% and lymphoma (PTLD) in 1.7%. As for solid organ malignancy, prostate, lung, cervical and renal origins account for the majority although any organ can be involved. Surgical resection of the malignancy is successfully done when early diagnosis is obtained. mTOR inhibitors may be beneficial with regard to possible less recurrence in a patient undergoing treatment for malignancy [18].

Renal dysfunction is not infrequent after transplantation. Not a few patients already have renal dysfunction to some extent due to long-standing low cardiac output. Antibiotic treatment for device-related infection in a patient on CFVAD may further deteriorate renal function. CNI has known side effect of renal dysfunction. Moderate grade of renal dysfunction (serum creatinine >2.5 mg/dl) is seen in 14.3% and hemodialysis is required in 6.0% within 10 years. Renal failure accounts for 8–9% of death 10 years and later after transplantation [1].

11.11 Demographics and Survival of Heart Transplantation

The annual number of heart transplantation reported to ISHLT registry is 5500—6000 recently [1]. This number is increasing in these couple of years due to mainly increase in the United States, caused by increased brain death by narcotics abuse and acceptance of HCV positive donors. There is a trend of increasing ratio of transplantation with ages of 60–69 years, 18.3% between 1988 and 1998 to 26.9% between 2010 and 2018. Ischemic etiology is decreasing and nonischemic dilated cardiomyopathy increasing (32 vs. 51% in 2018). BTT by using some type of mechanical circulatory support device accounted for over 50% recently, but will decrease due to UNOS policy change of allocation effective October 2018 (personal communication). Survival after heart transplantation is reported as 83.3%, 74.9%, 58.1%, and 41.3% at 1, 5, 10, and 15 years, respectively (Fig. 11.1).

The first heart transplantation was performed in 1999 in Japan after enforcing the brain death law in 1997. Annual number of transplantation was very limited (almost single digit) due to strict requirement of the law, but started to increase after revision of the law. Eighty-four transplantations were performed in 2019, and total number of transplantation reached 512 as of the end of 2019. According to the registry report by Japanese Society for Heart Transplantation [19], nonischemic dilated cardiomyopathy is a leading etiology accounting for 67%, followed by dilated-phase of hypertrophic cardiomyopathy in 11%, and post-myocarditis cardiomyopathy in 3.4%. Ischemic heart disease is only 2.0%. In recent years more than 90% of patients

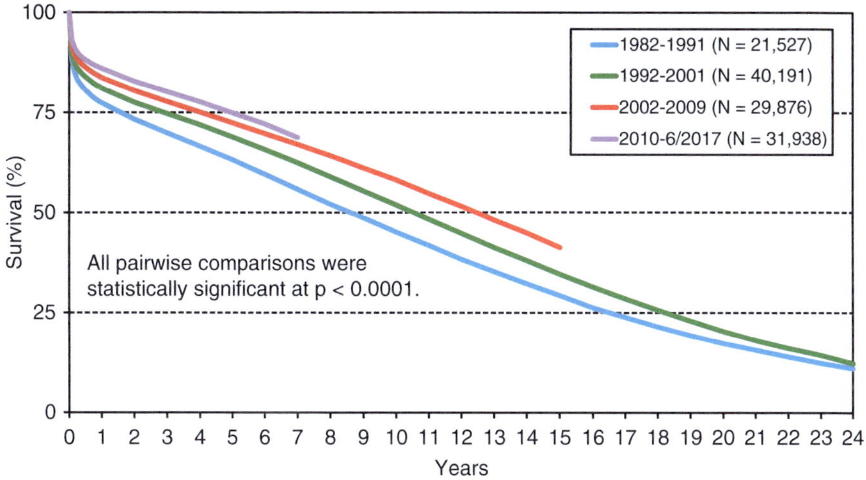

Fig. 11.1 Adult heart transplants—Kaplan–Meier survival by era (Transplants: January 1982–June 2017)

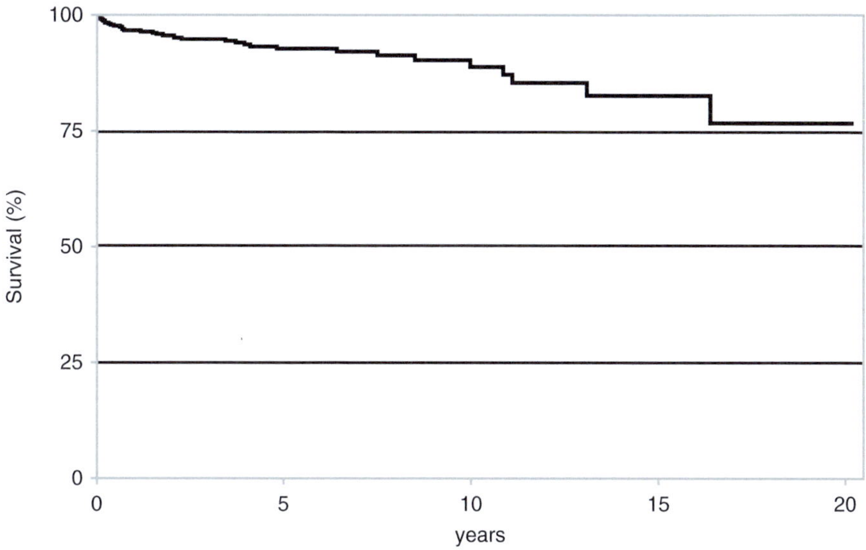

Fig. 11.2 Kaplan–Meier survival in Japan ($n = 476$)

reached to transplantation on a VAD support. Japan has 2 grade allocation system (Status 1 for patients on VAD or inotropic support and Status 2 for those with no support). Waiting period in Status 1 patients for heart transplantation has been lengthening and reached to 1310 days in 2018 [19]. Survival rate in 476 transplants by August 2019 is 96.7%, 92.8%, 89.8%, and 83.7% at 1, 5, 10, and 15 years, respectively, in Japan (Fig. 11.2).

References

1. Khush KK, Cherikh WS, Chambers DC, et al. The international thoracic organ transplant registry of the international society for heart and lung transplantation: thirty-sixth adult heart transplantation report – 2019; focus theme: donor and recipient size match. J Heart Lung Transplant. 2019;38(10):1056–66.
2. Billingham ME. Dilemma of variety of histopathologic grading systems for acute cardiac allograft rejection by endomyocardial biopsy. J Heart Transplant. 1990;9(3 Pt 2):272–6.
3. Dhital KK, Iyer A, Connellan M, et al. Adult heart transplantation with distant procurement and ex-vivo preservation of donor hearts after circulatory death: a case series. Lancet. 2015;385:2585–91.
4. Baumgartner WA, Reitz B, Kaper E, et al. Heart and lung transplantation. 2nd ed. Philadelphia, PA: WB Saunders; 2002. p. 57.
5. Miller LW, Kubo SH, Young JB, et al. Report of the consensus conference on candidate selection for Heart Transplantation-1993. J Heart Lung Transplant. 1995;14(3):562–71.
6. Mudge GH, Goldstein S, Addonizio LJ, et al. 24th Bethesda conference: cardiac transplantation. Task force 3: recipient guidelines/prioritization. J Am Coll Cardiol. 1993;22(1):21–31.
7. Fukushima N, Ono M, Saiki Y, et al. Registry report on heart transplantation in Japan. Circ J. 2017;81:298–303.
8. Kransdorf EP, Kittleson MM, Benck LR, et al. Predicted heart mass is the optimal metric for size match in heart transplantation. J Heart Lung Transplant. 2019;38:156–65.
9. Chang D, Kobashigawa J. The use of the calculated panel-reactive antibody and virtual crossmatch in heart transplantation. Curr Opin Organ Transplant. 2012;17(4):423–6.
10. Kitamura S, Nakatani T, Bando K, et al. Modification of bicaval anastomosis technique for orthotopic heart transplantation. Ann Thorac Surg. 2001;72:1405–6.
11. Stewart S, Winters GL, Fishbein MC, et al. Revision of the 1990 working formulation for the standardization of nomenclature in the diagnosis of heart rejection. J Heart Lung Transplant. 2005;24(11):1710–20.
12. Zuckermann A, Osorio-Jaramillo E, Aliabadi-Zuckermann AZ. mTOR inhibition and clinical transplantation: heart. Transplantation. 2018;102(2S Suppl 1):S27–9.
13. Costanzo MR, Naftel DC, Pritzker MR, et al. Heart transplant coronary artery disease detected by coronary angiography: a multiinstitutional study of preoperative donor and recipient risk factors. Cardiac transplant research database. J Heart Lung Transplant. 1998;17(8):744–53.
14. St Goar FG, Pinto FJ, Alderman EL, et al. Detection of coronary atherosclerosis in young adult hearts using intravascular ultrasound. Circulation. 1992;86(3):756–63.
15. Pazdernik M, Chen Z, Bedanova H, et al. Early detection of cardiac allograft vasculopathy using highly automated 3-dimensional optical coherence tomography analysis. J Heart Lung Transplant. 2018;37(8):992–1000.
16. Tona F, Osto E, Famoso G, et al. Coronary microvascular dysfunction correlates with the new onset of cardiac allograft vasculopathy in heart transplant patients with normal coronary angiography. Am J Transplant. 2015;15(5):1400–6.
17. Kobashigawa JA, Pauly DF, Starling RC, et al. Cardiac allograft vasculopathy by intravascular ultrasound in heart transplant patients: substudy from the everolimus versus mycophenolate mofetil randomized, multicenter trial. JACC Heart Fail. 2013;1(5):389–99.
18. Holdaas H, De Simone P, Zuckermann A. Everolimus and malignancy after solid organ transplantation: a clinical update. J Transp Secur. 2016;2016:4369574.
19. Registry Report of Heart Transplantation. From the homepage of Japanese Society of Heart Transplantation. http://www.jsht.jp/registry/japan/. Accessed 20 Feb 2020.

Chapter 12
Regenerative Medicine for Heart Failure: A Comprehensive Overview of Clinical Studies, Current Challenges, and Future Directions

Akifumi Matsuyama

Abstract Cell therapies have the potential to bring a paradigm shift to the treatment of heart failure (HF). Since the initial report of cell therapy with skeletal myoblasts in HF, a number of preclinical and clinical studies have been conducted, which support the ability of various stem cell populations to improve cardiac function and reduce the infarct size in HF. However, it is still too early in this new era of regenerative cell therapy as the novel modality. To address the fact that no cell therapy has been conclusively shown to be effective, the important issues involved have been discussed. First, the types of stem cells to be clinically investigated in HF have been reviewed; skeletal myoblasts, bone marrow-derived mononuclear and mesenchymal stem cells, adipose tissue-derived cells, and pluripotent stem cells have been discussed with their cell characteristics. Second, differentiation into cardiac lineage or paracrine effects as potential modes of action of stem cells in HF has been discussed. Finally, the routes of administration, cell dose and cell survival, and long-term engraftment have been discussed as current challenges and future directions. The purpose of this chapter is to review the preclinical and clinical studies carried out with respect to the use of stem cells in HF, and to discuss current unresolved issues and future directions.

Keywords Cell therapy · Skeletal myoblasts · Bone marrow-derived mononuclear and mesenchymal stem cells · Adipose tissue-derived cells · Pluripotent stem cells

---

A. Matsuyama (✉)
Department of Regenerative Medicine and Stem Cell Biology, School of Medicine, Fujita Health University, Toyoake, Aichi, Japan
e-mail: akifumi-matsuyama@umin.ac.jp

K. Kinugawa, T. Imamura (eds.), *Update of Non-Pharmacological Therapy for Heart Failure*, https://doi.org/10.1007/978-981-15-4843-7_12

12.1 Introduction

Heart failure (HF) is a common, but lethal, disabling, and expensive disorder. Despite the significant advancement in HF therapeutics, the prognosis for patients who are admitted to the hospital remains poor [1]. Although current therapeutics for HF improve symptoms and prolong life, the therapeutic approaches to regenerate cardiac tissues have been eager. It is for this reason that regenerative medicine with stem cells has generated great interest. Regenerative medicine with stem cells has the potential to dramatically transform the treatment and prognosis of HF with recovery of the loss of cardiac milieus. Stem cells were first applied in regenerative medicine in 2002 in patients with bone marrow cells [2]. Over the past 18 years, many clinical studies have been conducted that support the ability of various types of stem cells to improve cardiac function in ischemic and nonischemic cardiomyopathy, which is a main cause of HF. Despite this rapid advancement, no cell therapy has been conclusively shown to be effective in patients with HF. The purpose of this chapter is to review the clinical studies and trials conducted with respect to the use of stem/progenitor cells in HF in the clinical field, and to discuss current controversies, challenges, and future directions.

12.2 Stem Cell Types Clinically Investigated in HF

Stem cells are undifferentiated and self-renewing cells with a multi-lineage differentiation potential. Various types of stem cells have been tried for the treatment of HF (Table 12.1). Clinical studies have been employed for the use of stem cells in chronic HF.

Table 12.1 Stem cell types clinically applicable in HF

		Origin	Autologous	Allogenic
Pluripotent stem cells (PSCs)	Embryonic stem cells	Inner mass of blastocyte	×	○
	Induced pluripotent stem cells (iPSCs)	Somatic cells	○	○
Somatic stem cells	Skeletal myoblasts	Somatic cells	○	△
	Mononuclear cells	Bone marrow	○	○
	Endothelial progenitor cells	Bone marrow	○	○
	Mesenchymal stem cells	Bone marrow	○	○
		Adipose tissue	○	○
		Amnion	×	○
		Placenta	△	○
		Dental pulp	○	○

○: Applicable, △: Not recommend, ×: Non applicable

12.2.1 Somatic Stem Cells

12.2.1.1 Skeletal Myoblasts

Skeletal myoblasts are one of the somatic stem cell categories, and derived from satellite cells. As a skeletal muscle progenitor cell population, they are found under the basal membrane of myofibers of skeletal muscles. Because of their rapid expansion in vitro, skeletal myoblasts were the first cells to be translated into clinical studies in HF. The first human transplantation of myoblasts was performed by Menasche et al. in patients with severe ischemic HF [3]. Several studies showed augmented left ventricular (LV) function [3–6]. Based on the hopeful results of the studies, Menasche et al. conducted MAGIC, a phase II randomized, placebo-controlled, double-blind trial that examined the effects of intramyocardial injection of skeletal myoblasts plus coronary artery bypass graft (CABG) versus CABG alone as controls with severe HF and LV dysfunction [3]. Unfortunately, there were no significant differences in cardiac function between patients receiving myoblasts and the controls. Most of the results of the clinical studies and trials using skeletal myoblasts have encouraged researchers to promote regenerative medicine with skeletal myoblasts, but the MAGIC trial failed to confirm these findings. Many of these trials were performed in conjunction with CABG or LVAD (LV assist devise) procedures and the effects of myoblasts from those of revascularization or cardiomyocyte regeneration might not be differentiated from the patients who received injection of skeletal myoblasts to the controls. Because of the negative results of the MAGIC trial, the risk of arrhythmias, and the availability of other cell types, many researchers have given up the use of skeletal myoblasts clinically in cell therapy of HF. On the other hand, Sawa et al. have speculated that intramural injection of skeletal myoblasts into the cardiac parenchyma caused tissue damages, resulting in lethal arrhythmias. They have not given up, but introduced cell sheet technologies for cardiac regeneration. The first case was reported in 2012, in which a patient had severe HF due to dilated cardiomyopathy [7]. The case series of transplantation of skeletal myoblast cell sheet onto the surface of damaged LV anterior wall showed no lethal arrhythmia. The results made the team start the clinical trial for HF after designation as investigational new drug. Although all the cases did not show significant improvement of cardiac function after transplantation of skeletal myoblast-cell sheets, the approach showed suppressed exacerbation of HF in some cases. In 2016, HeartSheet® received a conditional and limited term biological license approval [8].

12.2.1.2 Mononuclear Cells Collected from Bone Marrow

Bone marrow is composed of many types of hematopoietic and non-hematopoietic cell populations. Due to the relatively greater amounts of stem cells in bone marrow and the ease and safety of procurement of these cells, a large number of clinical studies in HF have employed bone marrow-derived cells. Bone marrow mononuclear cells are a heterogeneous population composed of hematopoietic stem cells and endothelial progenitor cells, resident in bone marrow. As bone marrow can be easily procured with needle aspiration from patients, and mononuclear cells can be easily purified, and not required for cultivation, many researchers have started using them for preclinical and clinical investigations. The first clinical study was promoted by Perin et al. using autologous mononuclear cells in patients with chronic ischemic HF via transendocardial injection [9, 10]. A significant improvement in LV function and a reduction in end-systolic volume in cell-treated patients were reported after injection [9]. On the other hand, a number of studies using bone marrow-derived mononuclear cells in patients with ischemic HF failed to show efficacy [11, 12]. Additionally, trials using intracoronary infusion of mononuclear cells have been employed in patients with HF, and yielded mixed results. The TOPCARE-CHD study compared the effects of intracoronary infusion of circulating endothelial progenitor cells or mononuclear cells on LV function in HF, and showed that LV function improved significantly in patients receiving mononuclear cells, but not in those receiving circulating endothelial progenitor cells at 3 months after infusion [13]. However, other clinical trials have failed to present the efficacy of intracoronary infusion of mononuclear cells in HF [12, 14]. Studies of mononuclear cell administration in patients with chronic HF have shown mixed results like other small studies. Larger size trials are expected to attain manifest conclusions. Endothelial progenitor cells express CD34 on their surface as a typical surface marker, and could be mobilized from bone marrow into peripheral blood in response to ischemic injury, and promote neovascularization by differentiating into endothelial cells and re-endothelialization [15–17]. Autologous $CD34^+$ cell transplantation has been performed in patients with HF [18]. The initial experience with $CD34^+$ cells in HF was encouraging but limited by the small size of the trials.

12.2.2 Bone Marrow-Derived Mesenchymal Stem Cells

Mesenchymal stem cells (MSCs) are a subset of mesenchymal tissue-derived non-hematopoietic cells that are plastic-adherent under culture conditions. Bone marrow-derived MSCs (BM-MSCs) could be obtained from bone marrow, which was first reported by Pittenger et al. MSCs can differentiate into chondrocytes, adipocytes, osteoblasts, cardiomyocytes [19, 20], and endothelial cells [21]. The POSEIDON trial by Hare et al. proposed the effects of BM-MSCs in patients with HF [22]. In the study, both autologous and allogeneic BM-MSCs in patients with ischemic cardiomyopathy demonstrated improvement in LV function.

12.2.3 Adipose Tissue-Derived MSCs

Adipose tissue contains a pool of stem cells with multi-potency. From adipose tissue, stromal vascular fraction could be obtained after collagenase digestion, which contains endothelial cells, fibroblast, and stromal cells. From the heterogeneous stromal vascular fraction, stem cells could easily be obtained, which are designated as adipose tissue-derived stem/stromal cells (ADSCs) or adipose-derived MSCs (ADMSCs), and are able to replicate as undifferentiated cells, to develop as mature adipocytes. The preliminary results of the PRECISE trial indicated that administration of ADMSCs resulted in the stabilization of infarct size and improvement in maximal oxygen consumption [23]. However, there is no full report on adipose tissue-derived cells in HF. Moreover, adipose tissue-derived multi-lineage progenitor cells (ADMPCs) have been promising; they are a small population of stromal cells, which have higher differentiating capabilities than ADMSCs [24]. ADMPCs express SSEA-3/4 on their cell surface like pluripotent stem cells, as well as nuclear factors, *Nkx-2.5*, *GATA-4*, and *islet-1*, and could differentiate into cardiomyocytes, hepatocytes, and insulin-producing cells [24, 25, 26]. These reports have motivated researchers to conduct studies in animal models of HF. Using cell sheet technology, Shudo et al. reported that transplantation onto scarred myocardium of swine reversed wall thinning in the scar area and improved cardiac function [27], and they started the clinical studies for HF as an academic nonprofit IND in Osaka University in December 2019; the route of administration is epicardial spread with spray in conjunction with CABG.

12.2.4 PSCs

Pluripotent stem cells (PSCs) can be divided into two cell types: embryonic stem cells (ESCs) and induced pluripotent stem cells (iPSCs). ESCs are pluripotent cells harvested from the inner cell mass of preimplantation-stage blastocysts, and iPSCs could be reprogrammed from terminal differentiated cells with reprogramming factors. Although there are differences in their origins and establishing techniques, the pluripotent capabilities are similar to each other; they can form cell aggregates with floating cultivation and named embryoid bodies, with differentiating capacity to all three germ layers, ectoderm, endoderm, and mesoderm (including cardiomyocytes), and a lot of methods for differentiation into the cardiac lineage have been proposed [28]. PSCs-derived cardiomyocytes display adult cardiomyocyte morphology with properly organized sarcomeric patterns; they show spontaneous beating activity with characteristic atrial, ventricular, and nodal action potentials. The availability of hPSCs-derived cardiomyocytes has motivated investigators to research their effects in HF. In most studies on these cells conducted in a large animal model, cardiac-committed human PSCs have been transplanted onto infarcted myocardium, which improved LV function. Clinically, Menasche et al. reported that they grafted ESCs-derived cardiomyocyte-cell patches to severe HF patients [29], while Sawa et al. announced that they would start clinical studies using iPSCs-derived caridiomyocyte cell sheets [30]. Despite the well-examined cardiogenic capability of PSCs, biological hazards remain to be resolved. Because of their pluripotency, transplantation of hPSCs could be delayed by teratoma formation and tumorigenicity. Researchers know that only one teratoma or tumorigenic formation derived from PSCs-cardiomyocyte would be sufficient to halt clinical investigation of PSCs. It is promising that rapidly advancing technology in this field will overcome these hurdles, and ESCs and iPSCs-based approaches will be available for the therapy of HF.

Table 12.2 Potential modes of action of stem cells in HF

	Proposed mode of action
Replacement therapy	Cardiomyocyte differentiated from stem cells in vitro
	Vascular formation composed from administered stem cells
Paracrine or autocrine effect	Neovascularization
Cytokine therapy	Activation of intrinsic cardiac progenitor cells
	Anti-inflammation
	Fibrinolysis

12.3 Potential Modes of Action of Stem Cells in HF

The studies reviewed above suggest that some types of cells have shown improvement in cardiac function in chronic HF. What remains largely unknown, however, are the mechanisms responsible for these beneficial effects, in which regenerated cardiomyocytes could propose mechanical forces with beating and/or girdling effects, regenerated vasculature could supply blood flow, and/or fibrinolysis of the fibrotic scar in the infarcted myocardium. These various hypotheses proposed would be discussed (Table 12.2).

12.3.1 Differentiation of Cells into Cardiac Lineages

Cardiogenic differentiation of administered cells may occur. In a series of preclinical studies, somatic cells have been shown to differentiate into cardiomyocytes by in situ reprogramming [25]. However, the key issue is the number of resident cardiomyocytes derived from transplanted cells in cardiac milieu of patients with HF, and their participation in the improvement in function. In most of the preclinical studies, relatively small number of new cardiomyocytes is formed by differentiation of administered cells; consequently, the improvement of LV function cannot be accounted for solely by in situ reprogramming of the cells. Other mechanisms must be at work, and the supposed trophic action of paracrine effects, to date.

Recent advances have introduced to investigators that PSCs could differentiate into cardiac lineage, and PSCs-derived cardiomyocytes could be applicable clinically. Menasche et al. have reported that they applied ESCs-derived cardiomyocyte cell patches onto the injured heart of a patient with HF [29]. Sawa et al. have launched a clinical study with iPSC-derived cardiomyocyte cell sheets [30]. In the protocol, immunosuppressive agents will be administered for 3 months after transplantation, because they have reported that the transplanted cells could not survive for long term. In the preclinical studies, cardiomyocytes derived from PSCs have been reported; however, the cells showed beating but phenotype of immature cardiomyocytes. These results also remind us that PSCs-derived cardiomyocytes play a role in cardiac regeneration by the paracrine factors.

12.3.2 Formation of New Blood Vessels from Transplanted Cells

Formation of new blood vessels from transplanted cells has been observed in the cardiac milieu with various cell types in preclinical studies. This phenomenon is believed to be important in chronic myocardial infarction. Clinically, formation of new vessels may contribute to improved cardiac function in some patients with ischemic heart disease. In the setting of nonischemic cardiomyopathy, the phenomenon could not participate in the recovery of cardiac performance, because dilated cardiomyopathy might be affected in cardiomyocytes but not vasculature.

12.3.3 Paracrine Mechanisms

The paracrine hypothesis has been proposed to explain the beneficial effects of transplanted stem cells on the basis of their differentiation to noncardiac lineages [31], in which transplanted cells introduce myocardial repair by releasing bio-actives including autacoid, cytokines, chemokines, growth factors, and extracellular vesicles into the surrounding parenchyma. These bio-actives initiate and promote a sequential order of repair processes including activation of endogenous cardiac progenitor cells, neovascularization, inhibition of apoptosis, and favorable alterations of the extracellular matrix. Collectively, these actions result in enhanced LV performance, improved blood flow, and myocardial repair [31].

Activation of endogenous cardiac progenitor cells has been reported in preclinical studies. Injected cardiac progenitor cells and MSCs could promote the proliferation of endogenous cardiac progenitor cells in both the infarcted and non-infarcted regions, suggesting that paracrine-induced activation of the endogenous stock of cardiac progenitor cells was one of the modes of action in a rat model of chronic HF [32]. Cardiac progenitor cells have been known to secrete growth factors such as hepatocyte growth factor (HGF) and insulin-like growth factor (IGF-1) that stimulate other endogenous progenitor cells to proliferate and differentiate into cardiomyocytes, and reconstruction of vascular structures [33, 34].

MSCs can induce neovascularization by secreting chemokines such as stromal cell-derived factor-1 (SDF-1) [35–37] and angiotrophic factors such as vascular endothelial growth factor (VEGF), basic fibroblast growth factor (bFGF), HGF, IGF-1, and angiopoietin-1 [38–40]. EPCs could also secrete the endothelial and inducible isoforms of nitric oxide synthase (eNOS and iNOS), and promote proliferation of endothelial cells after recruitment to the ischemic area [41]. The resulting neovascularization and/or reconstruction of vasculature may improve blood supply to the viable cells that remain in the infarcted region, and thus improve LV function in HF. To date, there have been a number of reports in which neovascularization has been shown; however, there are no reports on the construction of neovascular network with arteriole, vein, and lymphatics. Supplementation and drainage of flow should be balanced after reconstruction of vasculature, or stiffness of LV wall would be increased, resulting in exacerbation of HF due to diastolic dysfunction of the heart.

Skeletal myocytes and MSCs have been reported to modulate various composition of the extracellular matrix, thereby causing LV remodeling and myocardial fibrosis. Skeletal myoblasts have been reported to remodel matrix collagen architecture [42], to reduce fibrosis in the peri-infarct and infarct-remote regions [43], and to modulate MMPs levels [38], suggesting a beneficial effect on remodeling of the extracellular matrix. Additionally, the deposition of massive extracellular matrix was reduced by ADMPCs via intracoronary infusion in a swine chronic myocardial infarction model [44].

12.4 Current Challenges and Future Directions

The clinical trials conducted to date suggests that administration of stem cells has a promising potential to improve cardiac function and regenerate viable cardiac parenchyma, resulting in the treatment of HF. To apply the potentials of stem cells in regenerative medicine to the full benefit of HF, there are a number of major unresolved issues that must be addressed. They include the route of administration, the cell dose, and the mode of action of each cell type. These issues can only be answered by careful discussion of the posted results of clinical studies and trials.

12.4.1 Route of Administration

Routes of administration of stem cells have been proposed (Table 12.3); however, the most effective one to deliver cells to the heart is still unknown. The major routes used to date have been direct injection into the LV wall via the endocardium or epicardium and intracoronary infusion. Transepicardial injection could be performed during cardiac surgery, CABG, and LVAD implantation [3]. However, needle injection of cells would damage the cardiac parenchyma and introduce arrhythmias, which have been observed in the MAGIC trials [45]. These unfortunate adverse events caused some people to promote cell patch technologies and HeartSheet®, which has been given a conditioned and limited term biological license approval by the Ministry of Health, Labor and Welfare, Japan. HeartSheet® can be transplanted onto the surface of injured heart directly without any other invasive operation [8]. Transendocardial injection could deliver cells directly into the LV wall by using an injection catheter. The advantages of this technique are that electromechanical mapping of the endocardial surface can differentiate viable, ischemic, and scarred tissues, thereby enabling targeted injection of cells into the border zone. There is a concern that intramyocardial injections may destroy tissue architecture and evoke cell clumps that disrupt adequate coronary flow, resulting in cell and tissue damages. Intracoronary delivery

Table 12.3 Routes of administration

Techniques of administration	Site of administration
Intramural injection as single cell or spheroid-suspension	Endocardial injection
	Epicardial injection
Put cell sheet/patch directly on the surface of heart	Epicardial injection
Spray directly on the surface of heart	Epicardial injection
Infusion as single cell-suspension	Intracoronary injection

of cells involves the infusion of the cells into a coronary artery. It has several advantages compared with transendocardial injection. First, it is a more uniformed distribution of cells within the infarcted region. Second, it does not require specialized training or a specialized equipment. Third, the technique is easier, and therefore more practical for utilization in the clinical field. However, intracoronary delivery also has certain disadvantages to transendocardial injection. Researchers wonder whether the retention level should be lower after intracoronary infusion than direct injection of the cells, presumably because of the rapid wash out of cells due to coronary flow, whether microvascular occlusion should occur when large cells are infused, and whether an occluded artery might prevent the delivery of cells to a targeted myocardial region. Practitioners should choose the route of administration in each patient based on the severity of HF, the status of stenosis or occlusion of coronary artery, and targeted LV regions in the future clinical field.

12.4.2 Cell Dose

It is obvious that the effects of cell-based therapies will depend on the number of cells administered; the doses of cells used to treat chronic HF have varied in the clinical studies and trials. It is one of the reasons why the results of the clinical trials cannot be compared easily. In previous reports, cell dose has been discussed from the viewpoint of efficacy. However, safety studies should be conducted in preclinical studies before promotion into the clinical studies and trials. In intramural injection of cells, total number of cells and cell density should be reviewed. Intramural injection could destroy the cardiac tissues; therefore, injection devises, number of injection sites, distance between each injection point, and the volume of each injection should be examined in preclinical safety studies with large animal models before promotion into clinical studies. Supposing cell patches or cell sheets would be applied onto the surface of the LV wall, the number of sheets should be of concern. Massive pile of cell sheets might prevent diffusion of oxygen, resulting in necrosis, which could evoke inflammation. There are also concerns that intracoronary infusion of cells might clog blood flow. Investigators assume that higher number of cells would deliver higher efficacy. The viable region of the LV wall can be affected by coronary infusion, resulting in microinfarction. Cell dose escalation studies should be conducted as preclinical safety studies with large animal models before promotion into clinical studies.

12.4.3 Cell Survival and Long-Term Engraftment

Regardless of cell type, dose, and mode of delivery, very low rates of cell survival and long-term cell engraftments have been suspected. To date, only the results derived from preclinical animal studies have been shown. In some reports, more than 90% of injected cells disappear in the first few days and less than 2% could still be found 4 weeks after transplantation [46, 47]. This massive cell loss is assumed to be due to the result of two sequentially distinct events. During or immediately after delivery, there is significant loss due to escape of cells via the coronary vein or leakage through intramural puncture holes coupled with removal through the venous system. Therefore, improving cell survival and engraftment is crucial to the progress of cell therapy in HF.

12.5 Conclusions

Cell therapies are a promising approach to HF treatment. The cell type to be administered and their specification, number of cells, route of administration, the formulation of cells such as single cells suspensions or cell patches remain unsolved and have been discussed in this chapter. It is important to remember that progress has been made in recent years, with acceleration. Many potential candidates for cell therapy have been examined in both preclinical studies with animal models and clinical studies with diseased patients with HF. During investigations, the favorable results of preclinical studies do not always promise efficacy in patients with HF in the clinical field. Large-sized, randomized clinical trials on HF have yielded heterogeneous efficacy outcomes, despite the potential results of case series or small-sized, non-randomized clinical studies. It is true that their efficacy and safety in HF has been unproven. The reasons include differences in too rapid translation despite a lack of comprehension of the specification of administered cells, their biological duties, and their precise modes of action. Their progress is now followed with both interest and fear. Future clinical trials should not only test safety and efficacy endpoints, but rather specific hypotheses on modes of action of efficacy. The cell type should be carefully selected and fully characterized in terms of specification, viability, function, optimal dose, and formulation of administered cells. The knowledge could then be applied in cell enhancement strategies. It would be surprising if a conclusive answer to these complex questions had been achieved in just a decade. However, with the encouraging results in these two decades, we believe that cell-based therapies are likely to become a clinical reality that may revolutionize the treatment of HF. We are now advancing into the clinical field of cell-based therapies for HF.

Acknowledgments The work discussed in this chapter was supported in part by the Grants-in-Aid and by the Highway Program for Realization of Regenerative Medicine from the Japan Agency for Medical Research and Development (AMED) to AM.

References

1. Stewart S, MacIntyre K, Hole DJ, Capewell S, McMurray JJ. More 'malignant' than cancer? Five year survival following a first admission for heart failure. Eur J Heart Fail. 2001;3:315–22.
2. Strauer BE, Brehm M, Zeus T, Kostering M, Hernandez A, Sorg RV, Kogler G, Wernet P. Repair of infarcted myocardium by autologous intracoronary mononuclear bone marrow cell transplantation in humans. Circulation. 2002;106:1913–8.
3. Menasche P, Hagege AA, Vilquin JT, Desnos M, Abergel E, Pouzet B, Bel A, Sarateanu S, Scorsin M, Schwartz K, Bruneval P, Benbunan M, Marolleau JP, Duboc D. Autologous skeletal myoblast transplantation for severe postinfarction left ventricular dysfunction. J Am Coll Cardiol. 2003;41:1078–83.
4. Ince H, Petzsch M, Rehders TC, Chatterjee T, Nienaber CA. Transcatheter transplantation of autologous skeletal myoblasts in postinfarction patients with severe left ventricular dysfunction. J Endovasc Ther. 2004;11:695–704.
5. Siminiak T, Fiszer D, Jerzykowska O, Grygielska B, Rozwadowska N, Kalmucki P, Kurpisz M. Percutaneous trans-coronary-venous transplantation of autologous skeletal myoblasts in the treatment of post-infarction myocardial contractility impairment: the Poznan trial. Eur Heart J. 2005;26:1188–95.
6. Herreros J, Prosper F, Perez A, Gavira JJ, Garcia-Velloso MJ, Barba J, Sanchez PL, Canizo C, Rabago G, Marti-Climent JM, Hernandez M, Lopez-Holgado N, Gonzalez-Santos JM, Martin-Luengo C, Alegria E. Autologous intramyocardial injection of cultured skeletal muscle-derived stem cells in patients with non-acute myocardial infarction. Eur Heart J. 2003;24:2012–20.
7. Sawa Y, Miyagawa S, Sakaguchi T, Fujita T, Matsuyama A, Saito A, Shimizu T, Okano T. Tissue engineered myoblast sheets improved cardiac function sufficiently to discontinue LVAS in a patient with DCM: report of a case. Surg Today. 2012;42(2):181–4.
8. Okada K, Miyata T, Sawa Y. Insurance systems and reimbursement concerning research and development of regenerative medicine in Japan. Regen Med. 2017;12:179–86.
9. Perin EC, Dohmann HF, Borojevic R, Silva SA, Sousa AL, Mesquita CT, Rossi MI, Carvalho AC, Dutra HS, Dohmann HJ, Silva GV, Belem L, Vivacqua R, Rangel FO, Esporcatte R, Geng YJ, Vaughn WK, Assad JA, Mesquita ET, Willerson JT. Transendocardial, autologous bone marrow cell transplantation for severe, chronic ischemic heart failure. Circulation. 2003;107:2294–302.
10. Perin EC, Dohmann HF, Borojevic R, Silva SA, Sousa AL, Silva GV, Mesquita CT, Belem L, Vaughn WK, Rangel FO, Assad JA, Carvalho AC, Branco RV, Rossi MI, Dohmann HJ, Willerson JT. Improved exercise capacity and ischemia 6 and 12 months after transendocardial injection of autologous bone marrow mononuclear cells for ischemic cardiomyopathy. Circulation. 2004;110:II213–8.
11. Hendrikx M, Hensen K, Clijsters C, Jongen H, Koninckx R, Bijnens E, Ingels M, Jacobs A, Geukens R, Dendale P, Vijgen J, Dilling D, Steels P, Mees U, Rummens JL. Recovery of regional but not global contractile function by the direct intramyocardial autologous bone marrow transplantation: results from a randomized controlled clinical trial. Circulation. 2006;114:I101–7.
12. Ang KL, Chin D, Leyva F, Foley P, Kubal C, Chalil S, Srinivasan L, Bernhardt L, Stevens S, Shenje LT, Galinanes M. Randomized, controlled trial of intramuscular or intracoronary injection of autologous bone marrow cells into scarred myocardium during cabg versus cabg alone. Nat Clin Pract Cardiovasc Med. 2008;5:663–70.
13. Assmus B, Honold J, Schachinger V, Britten MB, Fischer-Rasokat U, Lehmann R, Teupe C, Pistorius K, Martin H, Abolmaali ND, Tonn T, Dimmeler S, Zeiher AM. Transcoronary transplantation of progenitor cells after myocardial infarction. N Engl J Med. 2006;355:1222–32.
14. Yao K, Huang R, Qian J, Cui J, Ge L, Li Y, Zhang F, Shi H, Huang D, Zhang S, Sun A, Zou Y, Ge J. Administration of intracoronary bone marrow mononuclear cells on chronic myocardial infarction improves diastolic function. Heart. 2008;94:1147–53.

15. Kalka C, Masuda H, Takahashi T, Kalka-Moll WM, Silver M, Kearney M, Li T, Isner JM, Asahara T. Transplantation of ex vivo expanded endothelial progenitor cells for therapeutic neovascularization. Proc Natl Acad Sci USA. 2000;97:3422–7.
16. Rehman J, Li J, Orschell CM, March KL. Peripheral blood "endothelial progenitor cells" are derived from monocyte/macrophages and secrete angiogenic growth factors. Circulation. 2003;107:1164–9.
17. Krause DS, Fackler MJ, Civin CI, May WS. Cd34: structure, biology, and clinical utility. Blood. 1996;87:1–13.
18. Patel AN, Geffner L, Vina RF, Saslavsky J, Urschel HC Jr, Kormos R, Benetti F. Surgical treatment for congestive heart failure with autologous adult stem cell transplantation: a prospective randomized study. J Thorac Cardiovasc Surg. 2005;130:1631–8.
19. Pittenger MF, Mackay AM, Beck SC, Jaiswal RK, Douglas R, Mosca JD, Moorman MA, Simonetti DW, Craig S, Marshak DR. Multilineage potential of adult human mesenchymal stem cells. Science. 1999;284:143–7.
20. Toma C, Pittenger MF, Cahill KS, Byrne BJ, Kessler PD. Human mesenchymal stem cells differentiate to a cardiomyocyte phenotype in the adult murine heart. Circulation. 2002;105:93–8.
21. Reyes M, Dudek A, Jahagirdar B, Koodie L, Marker PH, Verfaillie CM. Origin of endothelial progenitors in human postnatal bone marrow. J Clin Invest. 2002;109:337–46.
22. Hare JM, Fishman JE, Gerstenblith G, DiFede Velazquez DL, Zambrano JP, Suncion VY, Tracy M, Ghersin E, Johnston PV, Brinker JA, Breton E, Davis-Sproul J, Schulman IH, Byrnes J, Mendizabal AM, Lowery MH, Rouy D, Altman P, Wong Po Foo C, Ruiz P, Amador A, Da Silva J, IK MN, Heldman AW, George R, Lardo A. Comparison of allogeneic vs autologous bone marrow–derived mesenchymal stem cells delivered by transendocardial injection in patients with ischemic cardiomyopathy: the POSEIDON randomized trial. JAMA. 2012;308(22):2369–79.
23. Perin EC, Sanz-Ruiz R, Sánchez PL, Lasso J, Pérez-Cano R, Alonso-Farto JC, Pérez-David E, Fernández-Santos ME, Serruys PW, Duckers HJ, Kastrup J, Chamuleau S, Zheng Y, Silva GV, Willerson JT, Fernández-Avilés F. Adipose-derived regenerative cells in patients with ischemic cardiomyopathy: the PRECISE trial. Am Heart J. 2014;168(1):88–95.
24. Okura H, Fumimoto Y, Komoda H, Yanagisawa T, Nishida T, Noguchi S, Sawa Y, Matsuyam A. Transdifferentiation of human adipose tissue-derived stromal cells into insulin-producing clusters. J Artif Organs. 2009;12:123–30.
25. Okura H, Matsuyama A, Lee CM, Saga A, Kakuta-Yamamoto A, Nagao A, Sougawa N, Sekiya N, Takekita K, Shudo Y, Miyagawa S, Komoda H, Okano T, Sawa Y. Cardiomyoblast-like cells differentiated from human adipose tissue-derived mesenchymal stem cells improve left ventricular dysfunction and survival in a rat myocardial infarction model. Tissue Eng Part C Methods. 2010;16:417–25.
26. Okura H, Komoda H, Saga A, Yamamoto-Kakuta A, Fumimoto Y, Lee C-M, Ichinose A, Sawa Y, Matsuyama A. Properties of hepatocyte-like cell clusters from human adipose tissue-derived mesenchymal stem cells. Tissue Eng Part C Methods. 2010;16:761–70.
27. Shudo Y, Miyagawa S, Ohkura H, Fukushima S, Saito A, Kawaguchi N, Matsuura N, Toda K, Sakaguchi T, Nishi H, Yoshikawa Y, Shimizu T, Okano T, Matsuyama A, Sawa Y. Adipose tissue-derived multi-lineage progenitor cells improve left ventricular dysfunction in porcine ischemic cardiomyopathy model. J Heart Lung Transplant. 2017;36:237–9.
28. Trounson A. A rapidly evolving revolution in stem cell biology and medicine. Reprod Biomed Online. 2013;27:756–64.
29. Menasché P, Vanneaux V, Hagège A, Bel A, Cholley B, Cacciapuoti I, Parouchev A, Benhamouda N, Tachdjian G, Tosca L, Trouvin JH, Fabreguettes JR, Bellamy V, Guillemain R, Suberbielle Boissel C, Tartour E, Desnos M, Larghero J. Human embryonic stem cell-derived cardiac progenitors for severe heart failure treatment: first clinical case report. Eur Heart J. 2015;36:2011–7.
30. iPS cell-based therapy for heart disease: clinical application iPS cell-derived cardiomyocytes. http://www.med.osaka-u.ac.jp/eng/archives/2777
31. Gnecchi M, Zhang Z, Ni A, Dzau VJ. Paracrine mechanisms in adult stem cell signaling and therapy. Circ Res. 2008;103:1204–19.

32. Tang XL, Rokosh G, Sanganalmath SK, Yuan F, Sato H, Mu J, Dai S, Li C, Chen N, Peng Y, Dawn B, Hunt G, Leri A, Kajstura J, Tiwari S, Shirk G, Anversa P, Bolli R. Intracoronary administration of cardiac progenitor cells alleviates left ventricular dysfunction in rats with a 30-day-old infarction. Circulation. 2010;121:293–305.
33. Rota M, Padin-Iruegas ME, Misao Y, De Angelis A, Maestroni S, Ferreira-Martins J, Fiumana E, Rastaldo R, Arcarese ML, Mitchell TS, Boni A, Bolli R, Urbanek K, Hosoda T, Anversa P, Leri A, Kajstura J. Local activation or implantation of cardiac progenitor cells rescues scarred infarcted myocardium improving cardiac function. Circ Res. 2008;103:107–16.
34. Hatzistergos KE, Quevedo H, Oskouei BN, Hu Q, Feigenbaum GS, Margitich IS, Mazhari R, Boyle AJ, Zambrano JP, Rodriguez JE, Dulce R, Pattany PM, Valdes D, Revilla C, Heldman AW, McNiece I, Hare JM. Bone marrow mesenchymal stem cells stimulate cardiac stem cell proliferation and differentiation. Circ Res. 2010;107:913–22.
35. Mathieu M, Bartunek J, El Oumeiri B, Touihri K, Hadad I, Thoma P, Metens T, da Costa AM, Mahmoudabady M, Egrise D, Blocklet D, Mazouz N, Naeije R, Heyndrickx G, McEntee K. Cell therapy with autologous bone marrow mononuclear stem cells is associated with superior cardiac recovery compared with use of nonmodified mesenchymal stem cells in a canine model of chronic myocardial infarction. J Thorac Cardiovasc Surg. 2009;138:646–53.
36. Askari AT, Unzek S, Popovic ZB, Goldman CK, Forudi F, Kiedrowski M, Rovner A, Ellis SG, Thomas JD, DiCorleto PE, Topol EJ, Penn MS. Effect of stromal-cell-derived factor 1 on stem-cell homing and tissue regeneration in ischaemic cardiomyopathy. Lancet. 2003;362:697–703.
37. Urbich C, Aicher A, Heeschen C, Dernbach E, Hofmann WK, Zeiher AM, Dimmeler S. Soluble factors released by endothelial progenitor cells promote migration of endothelial cells and cardiac resident progenitor cells. J Mol Cell Cardiol. 2005;39:733–42.
38. Shintani Y, Fukushima S, Varela-Carver A, Lee J, Coppen SR, Takahashi K, Brouilette SW, Yashiro K, Terracciano CM, Yacoub MH, Suzuki K. Donor cell-type specific paracrine effects of cell transplantation for post-infarction heart failure. J Mol Cell Cardiol. 2009;47:288–95.
39. Kinnaird T, Stabile E, Burnett MS, Lee CW, Barr S, Fuchs S, Epstein SE. Marrow-derived stromal cells express genes encoding a broad spectrum of arteriogenic cytokines and promote in vitro and in vivo arteriogenesis through paracrine mechanisms. Circ Res. 2004;94:678–85.
40. Gnecchi M, He H, Noiseux N, Liang OD, Zhang L, Morello F, Mu H, Melo LG, Pratt RE, Ingwall JS, Dzau VJ. Evidence supporting paracrine hypothesis for akt-modified mesenchymal stem cell-mediated cardiac protection and functional improvement. FASEB J. 2006;20:661–9.
41. Jujo K, Ii M, Losordo DW. Endothelial progenitor cells in neovascularization of infarcted myocardium. J Mol Cell Cardiol. 2008;45:530–44.
42. Farahmand P, Lai TY, Weisel RD, Fazel S, Yau T, Menasche P, Li RK. Skeletal myoblasts preserve remote matrix architecture and global function when implanted early or late after coronary ligation into infarcted or remote myocardium. Circulation. 2008;118:S130–7.
43. Fukushima S, Coppen SR, Lee J, Yamahara K, Felkin LE, Terracciano CM, Barton PJ, Yacoub MH, Suzuki K. Choice of cell-delivery route for skeletal myoblast transplantation for treating post-infarction chronic heart failure in rat. PLoS One. 2008;3:e3071.
44. Okura H, Saga A, Soeda M, Miyagawa S, Sawa Y, Daimon T, Ichinose A, Matsuyama A. Intracoronary artery transplantation of cardiomyoblast-like cells from human adipose tissue-derived multi-lineage progenitor cells improve left ventricular dysfunction and survival in a swine model of chronic myocardial infarction. Biochem Biophys Res Commun. 2012;425:859–65.
45. Eisen HJ. Skeletal myoblast transplantation: no MAGIC bullet for ischemic cardiomyopathy. Nat Clin Pract Cardiovasc Med. 2008;5:520–1.
46. Zeng L, Hu Q, Wang X, Mansoor A, Lee J, Feygin J, Zhang G, Suntharalingam P, Boozer S, Mhashilkar A, Panetta CJ, Swingen C, Deans R, From AH, Bache RJ, Verfaillie CM, Zhang J. Bioenergetic and functional consequences of bone marrow-derived multipotent progenitor cell transplantation in hearts with postinfarction left ventricular remodeling. Circulation. 2007;115:1866–75.
47. Hong KU, Li QH, Guo Y, Patton NS, Moktar A, Bhatnagar A, Bolli R. A highly sensitive and accurate method to quantify absolute numbers of c-kit+ cardiac stem cells following transplantation in mice. Basic Res Cardiol. 2013;108:346.

MIX
Papier aus verantwortungsvollen Quellen
Paper from responsible sources
FSC® C105338
www.fsc.org

If you have any concerns about our products,
you can contact us on
ProductSafety@springernature.com

In case Publisher is established outside the EU,
the EU authorized representative is:
Springer Nature Customer Service Center GmbH
Europaplatz 3, 69115 Heidelberg, Germany

Printed by Libri Plureos GmbH
in Hamburg, Germany